T0295231

THE PHARMACOLOGICAL GUIDE TO HALOPERIDOL

PHARMACOLOGY – RESEARCH, SAFETY TESTING AND REGULATION

Additional books and e-books in this series can be found
on Nova's website under the Series tab.

THE PHARMACOLOGICAL GUIDE TO HALOPERIDOL

AMOR HARLAND
EDITOR

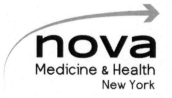

Medicine & Health
New York

Copyright © 2019 by Nova Science Publishers, Inc.

We have partnered with Copyright Clearance Center to make it easy for you to obtain permissions to reuse content from this publication. Simply navigate to this publication's page on Nova's website and locate the "Get Permission" button below the title description. This button is linked directly to the title's permission page on copyright.com. Alternatively, you can visit copyright.com and search by title, ISBN, or ISSN.

For further questions about using the service on copyright.com, please contact:
Copyright Clearance Center
Phone: +1-(978) 750-8400   Fax: +1-(978) 750-4470   E-mail: info@copyright.com.

Library of Congress Cataloging-in-Publication Data

ISBN: 978-1-53614-700-1
Library of Congress Control Number: 2018961871

Published by Nova Science Publishers, Inc. † *New York*

CONTENTS

PREFACE

Haloperidol is the most common neuroleptic drugs associated with a range of side effects caused by interactions with other drugs. In The Pharmacological Guide to Haloperidol, the authors review cases that report common pharmacodynamic and pharmacokinetic drug interactions of haloperidol *in vivo*.

Next, this compilation investigates methods for the determination of haloperidol in body fluids such as blood, urine and cerebral spinal fluid. Several techniques discussed include magnetic resonance spectroscopy, spectrophotometry and high performance liquid chromatography.

Also included is a description of haloperidol derivatives and their applications as antimicrobial agents, vasodilators and calcium channel blockers. Additionally, haloperidol derivatives that have potential applications for improving cardiac function and reducing oxidative stress are also addressed.

The authors present some studies which use functional magnetic resonance imaging to study aspects of haloperidol on facial expressions. Emotion processing is often notable in neurodegenerative diseases such as schizophrenia and evaluated in cerebral blood flow response in diseased patients.

The following chapter focuses on a literature analysis of the use of haloperidol, with studies indicating a potential limit for haloperidol efficacy; values above this limit don't appear to provide any supplementary clinical improvement.

Lastly, the authors provide a review of studies that have used magnetic resonance imaging to monitor haloperidol *in vivo*. Applications of 1H and 19F MRI in drug monitoring are discussed and a list of relevant studies is presented.

Chapter 1 - Haloperidol (4-[4-(4-chlorophenyl)-4-hydroxy-1-piperidyl]-1-(4-fluorophenyl)-butan-1-one) is the most common neuroleptic drug associated with a range of side effects due to interactions with other drugs. In this chapter, the authors will review cases that report common pharmacodynamic and pharmacokinetic drug interactions of haloperidol *in vivo*. The interaction of Haloperidol with lipids and Haloperidol-food interactions studied by biochemical and biophysical approaches are presented here.

Chapter 2 - The aim of this chapter is to investigate methods for the determination of haloperidol in body fluids such as blood, urine and cerebral spinal fluid. This chapter discusses the following techniques: reaction with 1,2-naphthoquinone-4-sulphonic acid, polarography, proton (^{1}H) magnetic resonance spectroscopy, spectrophotometry, high performance liquid chromatography, and gas chromatography with mass spectrometry (GC–MS).

Chapter 3 - Haloperidol and its derivatives are mainly used as antipsychotics, although other potential medical uses have been described in the literature. In this chapter, a description of haloperidol derivatives and their applications as antimicrobial agents, vasodilators, and calcium channel blockers are discussed. Additionally, haloperidol derivatives that have potential applications in improving cardiac function and reducing oxidative stress will also be addressed.

Chapter 4 - This chapter is presents studies using functional magnetic resonance imaging (fMRI) to study aspects of the drug haloperidol on facial expressions. Emotion processing is often notable in neurodegenerative diseases such as schizophrenia and evaluated in cerebral blood flow response in diseased patients during facial emotion. This chapter describes facial expressions, salient in emotional behavior, that are used in conjunction with (fMRI) to investigate emotion processing during schizophrenia treated by haloperidol. The applications of blood-oxygen-level-dependent (BOLD) techniques to study haloperidol responses and facial displays of emotions during haloperidol treatment are reviewed.

Chapter 5 - Functional magnetic resonance imaging (fMRI) has been used to probe brain biomarkers of healthy individuals and patients during haloperidol treatments. A current review is presented to examine the sensitivity of fMRI in behavioral testing performed for detecting early neurodegenerative changes related to all diseases treated by haloperidol. This chapter will also cover a literature analysis of the use of haloperidol, in which studies indicate a limit may exist for haloperidol efficacy; values above this limit seem not to provide any supplementary clinical improvement and may even reduce therapeutic effect.

Chapter 6 - In this chapter the authors will provide a review of studies that have used magnetic resonance imaging (MRI) to monitor haloperidol *in vivo*. Applications of ^{1}H and ^{19}F MRI in drug monitoring will be discussed. A presentation and list of recent studies using ^{19}F MRI for drug detection *in vivo* will also be presented. The authors' objective in this chapter is to provide reference information to the reader pertaining to the application of ^{1}H MRI, ^{19}F MRI, and fMRI to haloperidol monitoring.

In: The Pharmacological Guide to Haloperidol   ISBN: 978-1-53614-700-1
Editor: Amor Harland   © 2019 Nova Science Publishers, Inc.

Chapter 1

HALOPERIDOL INTERACTIONS

Dorota Bartusik-Aebisher, David Aebisher and Zuzanna Bober*

Faculty of Medicine, University of Rzeszów, Rzeszów, Poland

ABSTRACT

Haloperidol (4 - [4 - (4 - chlorophenyl) - 4-hydroxy – 1 - piperidyl] - 1- (4-fluorophenyl)-butan-1-one) is the most common neuroleptic drug associated with a range of side effects due to interactions with other drugs. In this chapter, we will review cases that report common pharmacodynamic and pharmacokinetic drug interactions of haloperidol *in vivo*. The interaction of Haloperidol with lipids and Haloperidol-food interactions studied by biochemical and biophysical approaches are presented here.

Keywords: fluorinated drug, haloperidol, drug-drug interaction

Very rapid progress in the field of pharmacology has resulted in the introduction of a large number of fluorinated drugs. Interactions are the

---

* Corresponding Author Email: dbartusik-aebisher@ur.edu.pl.

effect of one drug on the final effect of the second one used simultaneously.

- One of the medicines can:
- enhance or weaken the action of another drug
- shorten or prolong the operating time
- Mutual interaction of drugs, which the result is changes in their scope:
- absorption
- transport
- reducing or increasing the binding strength with blood and tissue proteins
- biotransformation and excretion

Depending on the mechanism such phenomena are distinguished: pharmaceutical interactions pharmacokinetic interactions and pharmacodynamic interactions.

In particular, Haloperidol may increase the neurotoxic effects of lithium carbonate. In rare cases, after the use of drugs containing lithium and haloperidol, a set of symptoms resembling encephalopathy (damage to the central nervous system) - disturbances of consciousness, confusion, headache, balance disorders and drowsiness. If you need to take Haloperidol together with lithium-containing medicines, your doctor should prescribe the least effective dose of Haloperidol and monitor your lithium levels. If you experience signs of encephalopathy-like syndrome, stop taking these medicines immediately. Haloperidol may inhibit the elimination of three-ring antidepressants. Below is a graph Figure 1 showing the number of Haloperidol interactions publications in the PubMed database.

While antipsychotic drugs are used for the treatment of schizophrenia, administering multiple drugs at the same time may counteract each other. Interactions are known to play a significant role in the incidence of adverse drug reactions (Table 1).

Table 1. Haloperidol interactions

Type of interaction	Factor	Reference
Haloperidol pretreatment dose-dependently potentiated the analgesic action of morphine and interfered with tissue morphine levels, potentiation of morphine analgesia by haloperidol is due, at least in part, to pharmacokinetic interaction	Interaction between morphine and haloperidol	Adamus et al. 1984
A 37-year-old woman with cerebral palsy and a rapid cycling bipolar affective disorder developed drowsiness and slurred speech	Interaction between haloperidol and carbamazepine	Brayley et al. 1987
21 days of 0.1 mg/kg haloperidol did not induce behavioral or biochemical tolerance. This finding is consistent with the lack of tolerance development to antipsychotic effects and suggests that animal models incorporating chronic low-dose neuroleptic regimens may be useful for the study of chronic treatment issues.	Haloperidol-amphetamine interactions and mesolimbic dopamine	Lynch et al. 1988
Behavioural and electoencephalographic interactions results demonstrate an interaction between dopamine and excitatory amino acid receptors	Interactions between haloperidol and PCP/sigma ligands in the rat	Sagratella et al. 1991
Vacuous jaw movements	Haloperidol interactions with scopolamine	Steinpreis et al. 1993
Groups treated with haloperidol exhibited heightened locomotion in response to cocaine and with repeated injections, showed a higher rate of behavioral sensitization than control animals	Interactions between haloperidol and cocaine	LeDuc and Mittleman 1993
The results from this study suggest that nefazodone has only modest pharmacokinetic and pharmacodynamic interactions with haloperidol.	Nefazodone and haloperidol interactions	Barbhaiya et al. 1996

Table 1. (Continued)

Type of interaction	Factor	Reference
Two weeks after the addition of fluoxetine, a very significant increase in haloperidol concentrations (more than 100 per cent) was noted; fluoxetine seems to have pharmacokinetic interactions with haloperidol, either by inhibiting its hepatic metabolism (inhibition of cytochrome P450 isoenzyme) or/and by displacing it from protein binding sites.	Interaction between fluoxetine and haloperidol	Viala et al. 1996
Findings confirm that fluoxetine impairs haloperidol clearance, this interaction is unlikely to have adverse clinical consequences, at least in patients chronically stabilized on a low dosage of haloperidol. As fluoxetine is a potent inhibitor of cytochrome P450 (CYP) 2D6, these results also provide indirect evidence for an involvement of CYP2D6 in the metabolism of haloperidol.	Interaction between fluoxetine and haloperidol	Avenoso et al. 1997
Lack of significant pharmacokinetic interaction	Interaction between haloperidol and grapefruit juice	Yasui et al. 1999
Biperiden reduced the serum haloperidol concentrations increased by the administration of carteolol. Adverse events of the central nervous system such as sleepiness and changes in pupil size were observed, but all were mild with clinical insignificance.	Interactions among haloperidol, carteolol hydrochloride and biperiden hydrochloride	Isawa et al. 1999
Results in decreased haloperidol blood levels	Interaction between haloperidol and carbamazepine	Cohen and Diemont 2002
Co-administration of haloperidol with nicotine, however, decreased memory performance compared with nicotine administration in isolation.	Nicotine interactions with haloperidol, clozapine and risperidone	Addy and Levin 2002

Type of interaction	Factor	Reference
The N-methyl-D-aspartate (NMDA) receptor antagonist, dizocilpine (MK-801), attenuated the cataleptic effects of haloperidol, but enhanced those of GHB.	Gamma-Hydroxybutyrate (GHB) interactions with haloperidol and dizocilpine.	Sevak et al. 2004
Drug interactions, when HP was associated with valerian, an increase in lipid peroxidation levels and dichlorofluorescein (DCFH) reactive species production was observed in the hepatic tissue in rats	Interactions between haloperidol and valerian	Dalla Corte et al. 2008
Increased significantly erythrocyte magnesium concentration	Interactions between magnesium and haloperidol	Nechifor 2008
Interaction of antipsychotic drugs with lipids	The effect of haloperidol (HAL), risperidone (RIS), and 9-OH-risperidone (9-OH-RIS) was examined on single lipid and mixtures comprising lipids of biological origin.	Alves et al. 2011
Molecular interactions	Affected by changes in the crystal habit of the drug molecule in haloperidol	Li Destri et al. 2011
Drug interaction	Drug-drug conditioning between citalopram and haloperidol or olanzapine in rats	Sparkman et al. 2012
Modulates midbrain-prefrontal functional connectivity in the rat brain	Dopamine D_2 receptor antagonists with haloperidol	Gass et al. 2013

Table 1. (Continued)

Type of interaction	Factor	Reference
Interaction with lipids	α-Lipoic acid interaction with dopamine D2 receptor-dependent activation of the Akt/GSK-3β signaling pathway induced by antipsychotics	Deslauriers et al. 2013
First, we administered haloperidol (0, 0.1 or 0.3mg/kg, ip) and found stronger catalepsy in rats with low reactivity to novelty. Second, we administered haloperidol (0.3mg/kg) or haloperidol plus nicotine (0.1mg/kg, ip) and found that nicotine indeed potentiated haloperidol catalepsy but only in rats with low reactivity to novelty.	Nicotine-haloperidol interaction	Boye 2013
Increased risk of psychosis and tardive dyskinesia	Interaction between haloperidol and dicyclomine	Vilar et al. 2013
Haloperidol treatment along with high, but not low, estradiol replacement was effective in reducing amphetamine-induced locomotor activity in sensitized rats. High estradiol treatment also augmented the effects of chronic haloperidol in reducing dopaminergic release in sensitized rats. These data suggest that estradiol levels affect both the behavioral and the dopamine responses to chronic antipsychotic treatment.	Estrogen has been shown to enhance the effects of antipsychotics in humans.	Madularu et al. 2014
Drug interaction	Haloperidol with Levodopa common pharmacodynamic drug interaction of haloperidol with levodopa in a 60-year-old female patient.	Lucca et al. 2015

Type of interaction	Factor	Reference
On brain volume changes in awake female rats.	To assess this interaction by investigating the effects of estradiol, AMPH and HAL	Madularu et al. 2015
Drug-to-drug interaction	Between voriconazole and haloperidol	Motta et al. 2015
Drug Interaction in modulating extrapyramidal motor disorders in mice	Interaction between anti-Alzheimer and antipsychotic drugs (Donepezil Galantamine and Haloperidol)	Shimizu et al. 2015
Drug release under gastrointestinal pH conditions	Haloperidol with water-soluble weak organic acids (malic, tartaric and citric acids) by using Neusilin® US2	Shah et al. 2015
Drug-induced parkinsonism	Methamphetamine and haloperidol	Matthew and Gedzior 2015
CYP2D6 *6/*6 genotype and drug interactions, severe iatrogenic extrapyramidal symptoms	CYP2D6 *6/*6 genotype and haloperidol interactions	Šimić et al. 2016
Central nervous system (CNS) depression and anticholinergic effect were the main possible effects of drug-drug interaction	Haloperidol and biperiden interactions	Ocaña-Zurita et al. 2016
Antipsychotic-nicotine interactions	Examined the specific drug-drug interactions between nicotine and haloperidol or clozapine in rats	Feng et al. 2017
Counteract each other, haloperidol could inhibit sucrase in non-competitive manner	Interaction of Antipsychotic Drugs with Sucrase	Jafari et al. 2017

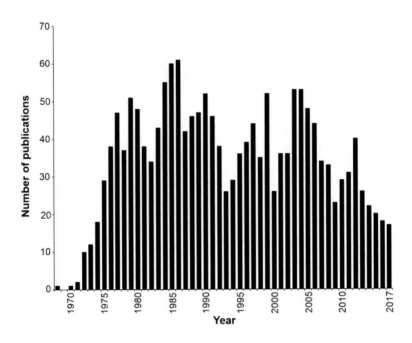

Figure 1. Number of publications on interaction of haloperidol collected from the Library of National Center for Biotechnology Information (NCBI) PubMed Data Base over the years starting from 1968.

Galphimine glauca can potentiate the cataleptic effect induced with Haloperidol (Santillán-Urquiza et al. 2018). Drug interactions are subject to drug - drug reactions amongst themselves, and with other psychotropics (Franken et al. 2016; Lucca et al. 2015; Madularu et al. 2015; Shah et al. 2015). *Aspergillus fumigatus* renal abscess treated with voriconazole following by haloperidol treatment showed an unexpected increase in voriconazole (Motta et al. 2015). Shimizu and coworkers examined the effects of cholinesterase inhibitors (Shimizu et al. 2015). Haloperidol induced focal changes in functional connectivity were found to be the most strongly associated with ascending dopamine projections which may reflect dyskinetic effects (Gass et al. 2013). Chronic administration of antipsychotics has been associated with dopamine D2 receptor upregulation and tardive dyskinesia (Boye 2013; Deslauriers et al. 2013). Present results indicate that drugs may change membrane compart-mentalization (Alves et al. 2011). Nicotine is capable of altering the long-term antipsychotic efficacy of haloperidol, while haloperidol can alter the behavioral effects of nicotine (Feng et al. 2017). Clozapine and nicotine are less likely to influence each other (Feng et al. 2017). Pharmacogenetics testing should be considered when drug toxicity is suspected, polymorphic metabolic pathways used and drugs concomitantly applied (Šimić et al. 2016). However, the pharmacological and behavioral mechanisms underlying drug-drug interactions in schizophrenia remain poorly understood (Sparkman and Li 2012). They also indicate that adjunctive citalopram treatment may enhance the antipsychotic efficacy of haloperidol and olanzapine in the treatment of schizophrenia (Sparkman and Li 2012; Li Destri et al. 2011). Della and coworkers suggest adverse interactions between haloperidol and valerian (Dalla Corte et al. 2008; Fang et al. 2001). Thus, genotyping may be useful for dose optimization with certain psychoactive drugs (Murray 2006; Zhang et al. 2005; Sevak et al. 2004). The effects of fluvoxamine on plasma concentrations of haloperidol and reduced haloperidol, and their clinical symptoms, in Haloperidol treated patients was reported (Yasui-Furukori et al. 2004). A pharmacokinetic interaction between haloperidol and carbamazepine results in decreased haloperidol blood levels (Cohen and Diemont 2002). These studies demonstrate interactions between nicotine and antipsychotic drugs in terms of memory, which may have important impacts on the treatment of schizophrenia (Addy and Levin 2002). Authors studied the interactive effects of the coadministration of haloperidol and chlorpromazine on plasma concentrations of haloperidol and reduced haloperidol showed a trend toward greater increases in plasma concentrations of haloperidol than those with other genotypes (Suzuki et al. 2001; Shin et al. 2001). Haloperidol, risperidone and olanzapine seem to have an equal effect on the gray matter cortical structure after 1 year of treatment (Crespo-Facorro et al. 2008). The aim of study conducted by Isawa was to investigate possible pharmacokinetic interactions of neuroleptic haloperidol with the beta-blocker carteolol and the anticholinergic biperiden (Isawa et al. 1999). The research shows that grapefruit juice does not affect the plasma concentrations of haloperidol (Yasui et al. 1999). The effects of smoking, on the steady state plasma concentrations of haloperidol and reduced haloperidol were evaluated (Pan et al. 1999). Aqueous solubility of haloperidol in presence of increasing concentrations of four different weak organic acids (malic, tartaric, citric, fumaric) were determined (Singh et al. 2013; Smesny et al. 2012; Billups et al. 2010; Giegling et al. 2010). Trifluoperazine and haloperidol could inhibit sucrase in non-competitive manner (Jafari et al. 2017; Delis et al. 2017). Drug-drug interaction must be considered when the patient with schizophrenia is medicated (Ocaña-Zurita et al. 2016). The extent and clinical significance of the pharmacokinetic interaction between fluoxetine and haloperidol was studied in 13 schizophrenic patients with prominent negative symptoms (Avenoso et al. 1997). Also no specific recom-mendations can be made, dosage adjustment may be necessary for haloperidol when coadministered with nefazodone (Barbhaiya et al. 1996). The additive effects of dopamine blockade by antipsychotics such as haloperidol (Matthew and Gedzior 2015). Haloperidol treatment along with high, but not low, estradiol replacement was effective in reducing amphetamine-induced locomotor activity in sensitized rats. (Madularu et al. 2014).

These results provide the first demonstration in rats that low levels of hormones can induce a pro-psychotic state that is resistant to at least typical antipsychotic treatment Arad and Weiner 2009; Bédard et al. 2013). Clozapine metabolism is complex and influenced by multiple factors, including interactions with hepatic P450 enzyme inducers/inhibitors, genetic polymorphisms and the potential for saturation of the N-demethylation metabolic pathway (Reznik et al. 2018; Almey et al. 2017; Vilar et al. 2013).

Findings have underlined the complex nature of potential interactions between dopamine receptors and brain peptidergic pathways, which have potential clinical applications (Palasz et al. 2016; Tatara et al. 2012; Tada et al. 2004).

Interventions by physicians and pharmacies have been developed to reduce the prescribing and dispensing of potentially harmful pairs of medications to patients with schizophrenia (Guo et al. 2012). Lipoic acid (LA) associated with ω-3 reduced the extrapyramidal effects produced by chronic use of haloperidol (de Araújo et al. 2017; Procyshyn et al. 2005; Hesslinger et al. 1999). Pharmacodynamic interactions of haloperidol, which may explain its analgesic efficacy, are summarized in paper by Colclough (Colclough et al. 2008). Psychotropic drugs (antidepressants, antimanic drugs, antipsychotics, analgesic opioids, and others) are among the most frequently used medicines. Between these drugs and magnesium there are pharmacokinetic and pharmacodynamic interactions (Nechifor 2008). Methodological issues are stressed, particularly drug plasma concentrations, dose-response relationships and time-course of effects (fluoxetine/buspirone), and unsolved questions are addressed (yohimbine/ caffeine, hydroxizyne/alcohol) (Barbanoj et al. 2006; Lerena et al. 2003). Clinical stability can be maintained with good tolerability during the transition from quetiapine monotherapy to periods of coadministration with haloperidol, risperidone, or thioridazine (Potkin et al. 2002; Hirokane et al. 1999). Examination of the stability of clonazepam, diazepam, alprazolam, haloperidol, respectively, along with an increase of lipophilicity (logP) from 2.12 to 4.30 for the most hydrophilic alprazolam to the most lipophilic haloperidol (Maślanka et al. 2013). Determinations of plasma and red blood cells concentrations of haloperidol and reduced haloperidol, and of fluoxetine and norfluoxetine, were conducted at the same time than clinical evaluations (Viala et al. 1996; Clement et al. 1994). This study was designed to evaluate the effects of a chronic treatment with the classical neuroleptic drug haloperidol on the preproenkephalin synthesis and its consequences for opioid and dopamine receptor-regulated adenylate cyclase in the developing and adult rat striatum (De Vries et al. 1994). The present series of experiments was conducted to investigate the vacuous jaw movements induced by sub-chronic administration of Haloperidol (Steinpreis et al. 1993). This experiment investigated the possibility that rats maintained on chronic haloperidol treatment would show increased behavioral responsiveness to cocaine, similar to that observed in human stimulant abusers who are chronically treated with neuroleptics. (LeDuc et al. 1993; Saha et al. 1991; Sagratella 1991). The moderate effect of CYP2D6*10 genotype on the pharmacokinetics and pharmacodynamics of haloperidol seems to be augmented by the presence of itraconazole pretreatment (Park et al. 2006; Michalets et al. 2000). A pharmacodynamic interactional study with omeprazole was undertaken in rats. Omeprazole (7 mg/kg, orally once daily for 14 days) significantly prolonged pentobarbitone (30 mg/kg, ip) induced hypnosis while it had no effect on haloperidol (1 mg/kg, ip) induced catalepsy or morphine (5 mg/kg, ip) induced analgesia models in rats. (Chandrashekhar et al. 1995). The antipsychotic drugs risperidone, paliperidone, olanzapine, quetiapine, aripiprazole, clozapine, haloperidol, and chlorpromazine have been reported to have various degrees of interaction (substrate or inhibitor) with the multidrug resistance transporter, P-glycoprotein (P-gp) (Reed et al. 2012). The use of antipsychotic drugs is limited by their tendency to produce extrapyramidal movement disorders such as tardive dyskinesia and parkinsonism (Murata et al. 2007). Apart from careful clinical observation, serum level monitoring of AEDs and psychotropic drugs can be useful in determining the need for dosage adjustments, especially if there is any change in seizure control, or possible toxicity (Spina and Perucca 2002). It is concluded that serum concentrations of reduced haloperidol are of minor value for the interpretation of data of therapeutic drug monitoring of haloperidol in patients with acute schizophrenia. (Ulrich et al. 1999; Lee et al. 1998). Haloperidol decanoate can be characterised by a flip-flop pharmacokinetic model because its absorption rate constant is slower than the elimination rate constant. Its plasma concentration peaks on day 7 after intramuscular injection (Froemming et al. 1989). The addition of ascorbic acid was not associated with any change in psychopathology in this group of patients, nor was there any apparent pharmacokinetic interaction with haloperidol (Straw et al. 1989). The use of anti-cholinergic drugs for counteracting neuroleptic induced extra-pyramidal side-effects is controversial. A possible increase in anticholinergic symptoms and a pharmacokinetic interaction are reported in literature (Altamura et al. 1986). The results indicate that the analgesic effect of morphine in the tail-flick test is correlated better with the spinal than cerebral morphine levels and that potentiation of morphine analgesia by haloperidol is due, at least in part, to pharmacokinetic interaction (Adamus et al. 1984). The biological half-life and other pharmacokinetic parameters of clinical importance are analyzed, and are used to predict steady-state levels and biological availability (Stafford et al. 1981; Forsman and Öhman, 1977). Haloperidol has been reported to undergo cytochrome P450 (P450)-mediated metabolism to potentially neurotoxic pyridinium metabolites; however, the chemical pathways and specific enzymes involved in these reactions remain to be identified (Avent et al. 2006; Iwahashi et al. 1995). These indirect effects of phencyclidine were also antagonized by haloperidol but not by reduced haloperidol. The data suggest that the metabolite, reduced haloperidol, is not an effective neuroleptic drug in the central nervous system (Kirch et al. 1985; Huang and Wilson 1984). This suggests that some patients who appear intolerant of carbamazepine may still benefit from this drug if concomitant haloperidol therapy is ceased (Brayley and Yellowlees (1987). Metabolic indices in this group suggested that increased DA availability partially competed with the neuroleptic receptor blockade in mesolimbic regions (Lynch et al. 1988).

CONCLUSION

We reviewed the interactive effects of co-administration of haloperidol and other drug on plasma concentrations of haloperidol and reduced haloperidol. The databases EBSCO, PubMed, ScienceDirect and SpringerLink are utilized to search the literature for relevant articles.

ACKNOWLEDGMENTS

Dorota Bartusik-Aebisher acknowledges support from the National Center of Science NCN (New drug delivery systems-MRI study, Grant OPUS-13 number 2017/25/B/ST4/02481).

REFERENCES

Adamus, A., Melzacka, M., Vetulani, J. (1984). Behavioral and pharmacokinetic interaction between morphine and haloperidol in the rat. *Polish Journal of Pharmacology and Pharmacy*, *36*:51-8.

Addy, N., Levin, E. D. (2002). Nicotine interactions with haloperidol, clozapine and risperidone and working memory function in rats. *Neuropsychopharmacology*, *27*:534-41.

Almey, A., Arena, L., Oliel, J., Shams, W. M., Hafez, N., Mancinelli, C., Henning, L., Tsanev, A., Brake, W. G. (2017). Interactions between estradiol and haloperidol on perseveration and reversal learning in amphetamine-sensitized female rats. *Hormones and Behavior*, *89*:113-120.

Altamura, A. C., Buccio, M., Colombo, G., Terzi, A., Cazzullo, C. L. (1986). Combination therapy with haloperidol and orphenadrine in schizophrenia. A clinical and pharmacokinetic study. *Encephale*, *12*:31-6.

Alves, I., Staneva, G., Tessier, C., Salgado, G. F., Nuss, P. (2011). The interaction of antipsychotic drugs with lipids and subsequent lipid reorganization investigated using biophysical methods. *Biochimica et Biophysica Acta (BBA) - Biomembranes*, *1808*:2009-18.

Arad M, Weiner I. (2009) Disruption of latent inhibition induced by ovariectomy can be reversed by estradiol and clozapine as well as by co-administration of haloperidol with estradiol but not by haloperidol alone. *Psychopharmacology*, *206*:731-40.

Avenoso, A., Spinà, E., Campo, G., Facciolă, G., Ferlito, M., Zuccaro, P., Perucca, E., Caputi, A. P. (1997). Interaction between fluoxetine and haloperidol: pharmacokinetic and clinical implications. *Pharmaceutical Research*, *35*:335-9.

Avent, K. M., DeVoss, J. J., Gillam, E. M. (2006). Cytochrome P450-mediated metabolism of haloperidol and reduced haloperidol to pyridinium metabolites. *Chemical Research in Toxicology*, *19*:914-20.

Barbanoj, M. J., Antonijoan, R. M., Riba, J., Valle, M., Romero, S., Jané, F. (2006). Quantifying drug-drug interactions in pharmaco-EEG. *Clinical EEG and Neuroscience, 37*:108-20.

Barbhaiya, R. H., Shukla, U. A., Greene, D. S., Breul, H. P., Midha, K. K. (1996). Investigation of pharmacokinetic and pharmacodynamic interactions after coadministration of nefazodone and haloperidol. *Journal of Clinical Psychopharmacology, 16*:26-34.

Bédard, A. M., Maheux, J., Lévesque, D., Samaha, A. N. (2013). Prior haloperidol, but not olanzapine, exposure augments the pursuit of reward cues: implications for substance abuse in schizophrenia. *Schizophrenia Bulletin, 39*:692-702.

Billups, J., Jones, C., Jackson, T. L., Ablordeppey, S. Y., Spencer, S. D. (2010). Simultaneous RP-HPLC-DAD quantification of bromocriptine, haloperidol and its diazepane structural analog in rat plasma with droperidol as internal standard for application to drug-interaction pharmacokinetics. *Biomedical Chromatography, 24*:699-705.

Boye, S. M. (2013). Individual phenotype predicts nicotine-haloperidol interaction in catalepsy: possible implication for the therapeutic efficacy of nicotine in Tourette's syndrome. *Behavioural Brain Research, 236*:30-4.

Brayley, J., Yellowlees, P. (1987). An interaction between haloperidol and carbamazepine in a patient with cerebral palsy. *The Australian and New Zealand Journal of Psychiatry, 21*:605-7.

Chandrashekhar, S. M., Chakrabarti, A., Garg, S. K. (1995). Pharmacodynamic interactions of omeprazole with CNS active drugs in rats. *Indian Journal of Physiology and Pharmacology, 39*:74-6.

Clement, R., Griff, D., Banks, B., Nemeroff, C., Kitabgi, P., Bissette, G. (1994). Effects of haloperidol, quinelorane, and lithium on regional neurotensin/neuromedin N concentrations: further evidence for neurotensin/neuromedin N-dopamine interactions. *Synapse, 17*:241-6.

Cohen, D., Diemont, W. L. (2002). Deterioration of schizoaffective disorder due to an interaction between haloperidol and carbamazepine. *Nederlands Tijdschrift voor Geneeskunde, 146*:1942-4.

Colclough, G., McLarney, J. T., Sloan, P. A., McCoun, K. T., Rose, G. L., Grider, J. S., Steyn, P. (2008). Epidural haloperidol enhances epidural morphine analgesia: three case reports. *Journal of Opioid Management*, 4:163-6.

Crespo-Facorro, B., Roiz-Santiáñez, R., Pérez-Iglesias, R., Pelayo-Terán, J. M., Rodríguez-Sánchez, J. M., Tordesillas-Gutiérrez, D., Ramírez, M., Martínez, O., Gutiérrez, A., de Lucas, E. M., Vázquez-Barquero, J. L. (2008). Effect of antipsychotic drugs on brain morphometry. A randomized controlled one-year follow-up study of haloperidol, risperidone and olanzapine. *Progress in Neuro-Psychopharmacology and Biological Psychiatry*, 32:1936-43.

Dalla Corte, C. L., Fachinetto, R., Colle, D., Pereira, R. P., Avila, D. S., Villarinhom J. G., Wagner, C., Pereira, M. E., Nogueira, C. W., Soares, F. A., Rocha, J. B. (2008). Potentially adverse interactions between haloperidol and valerian. *Food and Chemical Toxicology: an International Journal Published for the British Industrial Biological Research Association*, 46:2369-75.

de Araújo, D. P., Camboim, T. G. M., Silva, A. P. M., Silva, C. D. F., de Sousa, R. C., Barbosa, M. D. A., Oliveira, L. C., Cavalcanti, J. R. L. P., Lucena, E. E. S., Guzen, F. P. (2017). Behavioral and neurochemical effects of alpha lipoic acid associated with omega-3 in tardive dyskinesia induced by chronic haloperidol in rats. *Canadian Journal of Physiology and Pharmacology*, 95:837-843.

De Vries, T. J., Jonker, A. J., Voorn, P., Mulder, A. H., Schoffelmeer, A. N. (1994). Adaptive changes in rat striatal preproenkephalin expression and dopamine-opioid interactions upon chronic haloperidol treatment during different developmental stages. *Brain Research. Developmental Brain Research*, 78:175-81.

Delis, F., Rosko, L., Shroff, A., Leonard, K. E., Thanos, P. K. (2017). Oral haloperidol or olanzapine intake produces distinct and region-specific increase in cannabinoid receptor levels that is prevented by high fat diet. *Progress in Neuro-Psychopharmacology & Biological Psychiatry.*, 79:268-80.

Deslauriers, J., Desmarais, C., Sarret, P., Grignon, S. (2013). α-Lipoic acid interaction with dopamine D2 receptor-dependent activation of the Akt/GSK-3β signaling pathway induced by antipsychotics: potential relevance for the treatment of schizophrenia. *Journal of Molecular Neuroscience*, *50*:134-45.

Fang, J., McKay, G., Song, J., Remillrd, A., Li, X., Midha, K. (2001). *In vitro* characterization of the metabolism of haloperidol using recombinant cytochrome P450 enzymes and human liver microsomes. *Drug Metabolism and Disposition*, *29*:1638-43.

Feng, M., Sparkman, N. L., Sui, N., Li, M. (2017). A drug-drug conditioning paradigm reveals multiple antipsychotic-nicotine interactions. *Journal of Psychopharmacology*, *31*:474-86.

Forsman, A., Öhman, R. (1977). Applied pharmacokinetics of haloperidol in man. *Current Therapeutic Research*, *21*(3), 396-411.

Franken, L. G., de Winter, B. C., van Esch, H. J., van Zuylen, L., Baar, F. P., Tibboel, D., Mathôt, R. A., van Gelder, T., Koch, B. C. (2016). Pharmacokinetic considerations and recommendations in palliative care, with focus on morphine, midazolam and haloperidol. *Expert Opinion in Drug Metabolic Toxicology*, *12*:669-80.

Froemming, J. S., Lam, Y. W., Jann, M. W., Davis, C. M. (1989). Pharmacokinetics of haloperidol. *Clinical Pharmacokinetics*, *17*:396-423.

Gass, N., Schwarz, A. J., Sartorius, A., Cleppien, D., Zheng, L., Schenker, E., Risterucci, C., Meyer-Lindenberg, A., Weber-Fahr, W. (2013). Haloperidol modulates midbrain-prefrontal functional connectivity in the rat brain. *European Neuropsychopharmacology: The Journal of the European College of Neuropsychopharmacology*, *23*:1310-9.

Giegling, I., Drago, A., Schäfer, M., Möller, H. J., Rujescu, D., Serretti, A. (2010). Interaction of haloperidol plasma level and antipsychotic effect in early phases of acute psychosis treatment. *Journal of Psychiatric Research*, *44*:487-92.

Gorrod, J. W., Fang, J. (1993). On the metabolism of haloperidol. *Xenobiotica; the Fate of Foreign Compounds in Biological Systems*, *23*:495-508.

Guo, J. J., Wu, J., Kelton, C. M., Jing, Y., Fan, H., Keck, P. E., Patel, N. C. (2012). Exposure to potentially dangerous drug-drug interactions involving antipsychotics. *Psychiatric services: a Journal of the American Psychiatric Association*, *63*:1080-8.

Hesslinger, B., Normann, C., Langosch, J. M., Klose, P., Berger, M., Walden, J. (1999). Effects of carbamazepine and valproate on haloperidol plasma levels and on psychopathologic outcome in schizophrenic patients. *Journal of Clinical Psychopharmacology*, *19*:310-5.

Hirokane, G., Someya, T., Takahashi, S., Morita, S., Shimoda, K. (1999). Interindividual variation of plasma haloperidol concentrations and the impact of concomitant medications: the analysis of therapeutic drug monitoring data. *Therapeutic Drug Monitoring*, *21*:82-6.

Huang, D., Wilson, M. C. (1984). The effects of dl-cathinone, d-amphetamine and cocaine on avoidance responding in rats and their interactions with haloperidol and methysergide. *Pharmacology, Biochemistry, and Behawior*, *20*:721-9.

Isawa, S., Murasaki, M., Miura, S., Yoshioka, M., Uchiumi, M., Kumagai, Y., Aoki, S., Hisazumi, H., Kudo, S. (1999). Pharmacokinetic and pharmacodynamic interactions among haloperidol, carteolol hydrochloride and biperiden hydrochloride. *Japanese Journal of Psychopharmacology*, *19*(3):111-8.

Iwahashi, K., Miyatake, R., Suwaki, H., Hosokawa, K., Ichikawa, Y. (1995). The drug-drug interaction effects of haloperidol on plasma carbamazepine levels. *Clinical Neuropharmacology*, *18*(3):233-6.

Iwahashi, K., Miyatake, R., Suwaki, H., Hosokawa, K., Ichikawa, Y. (1995). The drug-drug interaction effects of haloperidol on plasma carbamazepine levels. *Clinical Neuropharmacology*, *18*(3):233-6.

Jafari, N., Dehganpour, H., Ghavanini, N., Mollasalehi, H., Minai-Tehrani, D. (2017). Interaction of Antipsychotic Drugs with Sucrase, Kinetics and Structural Study. *Current Clinical Pharmacology*, *12*:50-4.

Kirch, D. G., Palmer, M. R., Egan, M., Freedman, R. (1985). Electrophysiological interactions between haloperidol and reduced haloperidol, and dopamine, norepinephrine and phencyclidine in rat brain. *Neuropharmacology, 24*:375-9.

LeDuc, P. A., Mittleman, G. (1993). Interactions between chronic haloperidol treatment and cocaine in rats: an animal model of intermittent cocaine use in neuroleptic treated populations. *Psychopharmacology, 110*:427-36.

Lee, M. S., Kim, Y. K., Lee, S. K., Suh, K. Y. (1998). A double-blind study of adjunctive sertraline in haloperidol-stabilized patients with chronic schizophrenia. *Journal of Clinical Psychopharmacology, 18*:399-403.

Li Destri, G., Marrazzo, A., Rescifina, A., Punzo, F. (2011). How molecular interactions affect crystal morphology: the case of haloperidol. *Journal of Pharmaceutical Sciences, 100*:4896-906.

LLerena, A., Berecz, R., Dorado, P., de la Garza, C. S., Norberto, M. J., Cáceres, M., Gutiérrez, J. R. (2003). Determination of risperidone and 9-hydroxyrisperidone in human plasma by liquid chromatography: application to the evaluation of CYP2D6 drug interactions. *Journal of Chromatography. B, Analytical Technologies in the Biomedical and Life Sciences, 783*:213-9.

Lucca, J. M., Ramesh, M., Parthasarathi, G., Raman, R. (2015). An adverse drug interaction of haloperidol with levodopa. *Indian journal of psychological medicine, 37*:220-2.

Lynch, M. R., Kuhn, H. G., Carey, R. J. (1988). Chronic haloperidol-amphetamine interactions and mesolimbic dopamine. *Neuropsychobiology, 19*:97-103.

Madularu, D., Kulkarni, P., Ferris, C. F., Brake, W. G. (2015). Changes in brain volume in response to estradiol levels, amphetamine sensitization and haloperidol treatment in awake female rats. *Brain Research, 1618*:100-10.

Madularu, D., Shams, W. M., Brake, W. G. (2014). Estrogen potentiates the behavioral and nucleus accumbens dopamine response to continuous haloperidol treatment in female rats. *The European Journal of Neuroscience, 39*:257-65

Maślanka, A., Krzek, J., Szlósarczyk, M., Żmudzki, P., Wach, K. (2013). Dependence of the kinetic and thermodynamic parameters on hydrophilic-lipophilic character of alprazolam, clonazepam, diazepam, doxepin and haloperidol in alkaline environment. *International Journal of Pharmaceutics, 455*:104-12.

Matthew, B. J., Gedzior, J. S. (2015). Drug-induced Parkinsonism following chronic methamphetamine use by a patient on haloperidol decanoate. *International Journal of Psychiatry in Medicine, 50*:405-11.

Michalets, E. L., Williams, C. R. (2000). Drug interactions with cisapride: clinical implications. *Clinical Pharmacokinetics, 39*:49-75.

Motta, I., Calcagno, A., Baietto, L., D'Avolio, A., De Rosa, F. G., Bonora, S. (2015). A probable drug-to-drug interaction between voriconazole and haloperidol in a CYP2C19 poor metabolizing patient. *Le Infezioni in Medicina: Rivista Periodica di Eziologia, Epidemiologia, Diagnostica, Clinica e Terapia Delle Patologie Infettive, 23*:367-9.

Murata, T., Maruoka, N., Omata, N., Takashima, Y., Igarashi, K., Kasuya, F., Fujibayashi, Y., Wada, Y. (2007). Effects of haloperidol and its pyridinium metabolite on plasma membrane permeability and fluidity in the rat brain. *Progress in Neuro-Psychopharmacology & Biological Psychiatry, 31*:848-57.

Murray, M. (2006). Role of CYP pharmacogenetics and drug-drug interactions in the efficacy and safety of atypical and other antipsychotic agents. *The Journal of Pharmacy and Pharmacology, 58*:871-85.

Nechifor M. (2008). Interactions between magnesium and psychotropic drugs. *Magnesium Research, 21*:97-100.

Ocaña-Zurita, M. C., Juárez-Rojop, I. E., Genis, A., Tovilla-Zárate, C. A., González-Castro, T. B., Lilia López-Narváez, M., de la O de la O, M. E., Nicolini, H. (2016). Potential drug-drug interaction in Mexican patients with schizophrenia. *International Journal of Psychiatry in Clinical Practice, 20*:249-53.

Palasz, A., Rojczyk, E., Golyszny, M., Filipczyk, L., Worthington, J. J., Wiaderkiewicz, R. (2016). Long-term treatment with haloperidol affects neuropeptide S and NPSR mRNA levels in the rat brain. *Acta Neuropsychiatrica, 28*:110-6.

Pan, L., Vander Stichele, R., Rosseel, M. T., Berlo, J. A., De Schepper, N., Belpaire, F. M. (1999). Effects of smoking, CYP2D6 genotype, and concomitant drug intake on the steady state plasma concentrations of haloperidol and reduced haloperidol in schizophrenic inpatients. *Therapeutic Drug Monitoring, 21*(5):489-97.

Park, J. Y., Shon, J. H., Kim, K. A., Jung, H. J., Shim, J. C., Yoon, Y. R., Cha, I. J., Shin, J. G. (2006). Combined effects of itraconazole and CYP2D6*10 genetic polymorphism on the pharmacokinetics and pharmacodynamics of haloperidol in healthy subjects. *Journal of Clinical Psychopharmacology, 26*:135-42.

Potkin, S. G., Thyrum, P. T., Alva, G., Bera, R., Yeh, C., Arvanitis, L. A. (2002). The safety and pharmacokinetics of quetiapine when coadministered with haloperidol, risperidone, or thioridazine. *Journal of Clinical Psychopharmacology, 22*:121-30.

Reed, A., Huie, K., Perloff, E. S., Cassella, J. V., Takahashi, L. H. (2012). Loxapine P-glycoprotein interactions *in vitro*. *Drug Metabolism Letters, 6*:26-32.

Sagratella, S., Scotti de Carolis, A., Pèzzola, A., Popoli, P. (1991). Behavioural and electoencephalographic interactions between haloperidol and PCP/sigma ligands in the rat. *Psychopharmacology, 105*:485-91.

Saha, N., Datta, H., Sharma, P. L. (1991). Effects of morphine on memory: interactions with naloxone, propranolol and haloperidol. *Pharmacology, 42*:10-4.

Santillán-Urquiza, M. A., Herrera-Ruiz, M., Zamilpa, A., Jiménez-Ferrer, E., Román-Ramos, R., Tortoriello, J. (2018). Pharmacological interaction of Galphimia glauca extract and natural galphimines with Ketamine and Haloperidol on different behavioral tests. *Biomedicine & Pharmacotherapy, 103*:879-88.

Sevak, R. J., France, C. P., Koek, W. (2004). Neuroleptic-like effects of gamma-hydroxybutyrate: interactions with haloperidol and dizocilpine. *European Journal of Pharmacology, 483*:289-93.

Shah, A., Serajuddin, A. T. (2015). Conversion of solid dispersion prepared by acid-base interaction into free-flowing and table powder by using Neusilin® US2. *International Journal of Pharmaceutics*, *484*:172-80.

Shimizu, S., Mizuguchi, Y., Sobue, A., Fujiwara, M., Morimoto, T., Ohno, Y. (2015). Interaction between anti-Alzheimer and antipsychotic drugs in modulating extrapyramidal motor disorders in mice. *Journal of Pharmacological Sciences*, *127*:439-45.

Shin, J. G., Kane, K., Flockhart, D. A. (2001). Potent inhibition of CYP2D6 by haloperidol metabolites: stereoselective inhibition by reduced haloperidol. *British Journal of Clinical Pharmacology*, *51*: 45-52.

Šimić, I., Potočnjak, I., Kraljičković, I., Stanić Benić, M., Čegec, I., Juričić Nahal, D., Ganoci, L., Božina, N. (2016). CYP2D6 *6/*6 genotype and drug interactions as cause of haloperidol-induced extrapyramidal symptoms. *Pharmacogenomics*, *17*:1385-9.

Singh, S., Parikh, T., Sandhu, H. K., Shah, N. H., Malick, A. W., Singhal, D., Serajuddin, A. T. (2013). Supersolubilization and amorphization of a model basic drug, haloperidol, by interaction with weak acids. *Pharmaceutical Research*, *30*:1561-73.

Smesny, S., Langbein, K., Rzanny, R., Gussew, A., Burmeister, H. P., Reichenbach, J. R., Sauer, H. (2012). Antipsychotic drug effects on left prefrontal phospholipid metabolism: a follow-up 31P-2D-CSI study of haloperidol and risperidone in acutely ill chronic schizophrenia patients. *Schizophrenia Research*, *138*:164-70.

Sparkman, N. L., Li, M. (2012). Drug-drug conditioning between citalopram and haloperidol or olanzapine in a conditioned avoidance response model: implications for polypharmacy in schizophrenia. *Behavioural Pharmacology*, *23*:658-68.

Spina, E., Perucca E. (2002). Clinical significance of pharmacokinetic interactions between antiepileptic and psychotropic drugs. *Epilepsia*, *43*:37-44.

Stafford, J. E., Jackson, L. S., Forrest, T. J., Barrow, A., Palmer, R. F. (1981). Haloperidol pharmacokinetics: a preliminary study in rhesus monkeys using a new radioimmunoassay procedure. *Journal of Pharmacological Methods*, 6:261-79.

Steinpreis, R. E., Baskin, P., Salamone, J. D. (1993). Vacuous jaw movements induced by sub-chronic administration of haloperidol: interactions with scopolamine. *Psychopharmacology*, *111*:99-105.

Straw, G. M., Bigelow, L. B., Kirch, D. G. (1989). Haloperidol and reduced haloperidol concentrations and psychiatric ratings in schizophrenic patients treated with ascorbic acid. *Journal of Clinical Psychopharmacology*, 9(2):130-2.

Suzuki, Y., Someya, T., Shimoda, K., Hirokane, G., Morita, S., Yokono, A., Inoue, Y., Takahashi, S. (2001). Importance of the cytochrome P450 2D6 genotype for the drug metabolic interaction between chlorpromazine and haloperidol. *Therapeutic Drug Monitoring*, *23*:363-8.

Swalve, N., Li, M. (2012). Parametric studies of antipsychotic-induced sensitization in the conditioned avoidance response model: roles of number of drug exposure, drug dose, and test-retest interval. *Behavioural Pharmacology*, *23*:380-91.

Tada, M., Shirakawa, K., Matsuoka, N., Mutoh, S. (2004). Combined treatment of quetiapine with haloperidol in animal models of antipsychotic effect and extrapyramidal side effects: comparison with risperidone and chlorpromazine. *Psychopharmacology*, *176*:94-100.

Tatara, A., Shimizu, S., Shin, N., Sato, M., Sugiuchi, T., Imaki, J., Ohno, Y. (2012). Modulation of antipsychotic-induced extrapyramidal side effects by medications for mood disorders. *Progress in Neuro-Psychopharmacology & Biological Psychiatry*, *38*:252-9.

Ulrich, S., Neuhof, S., Braun, V., Meyer, F. P. (1999). Reduced haloperidol does not interfere with the antipsychotic activity of haloperidol in the treatment of acute schizophrenia. *International Clinical Psychopharmacology*, *14*:219-28.

Viala, A., Aymard, N., Leyris, A., Caroli, F. (1996). Pharmaco-clinical correlations during fluoxetine administration in patients with depressive schizophrenia treated with haloperidol decanoate. *Therapie*, *51*:19-25.

Vilar, S., Uriarte, E., Santana, L., Tatonetti, N. P., Friedman, C. (2013). Detection of drug-drug interactions by modeling interaction profile fingerprints. *PLoS One*, *8*:e58321.

Yasui, N., Kondo, T., Suzuki, A., Otani, K., Mihara, K., Furukori, H., Kaneko, S., Inoue, Y. (1999). Lack of significant pharmacokinetic interaction between haloperidol and grapefruit juice. *International Clinical Psychopharmacology.*, *14*:113-8.

Yasui-Furukori, N., Kondo, T., Mihara, K., Inoue, Y., Kaneko, S. (2004). Fluvoxamine dose-dependent interaction with haloperidol and the effects on negative symptoms in schizophrenia. *Psychopharmacology (Berl)*, *171*:223-7.

Zhang, M., Ballard, M. E., Pan, L., Roberts, S., Faghih, R., Cowart, M., Esbenshade, T. A., Fox, G. B., Decker, M. W., Hancock, A. A., Rueter, L. E. (2005). Lack of cataleptogenic potentiation with non-imidazole H3 receptor antagonists reveals potential drug-drug interactions between imidazole-based H3 receptor antagonists and antipsychotic drugs. *Brain Research*, *1045*:142-9.

In: The Pharmacological Guide to Haloperidol   ISBN: 978-1-53614-700-1
Editor: Amor Harland   © 2019 Nova Science Publishers, Inc.

Chapter 2

DETERMINATIONS OF HALOPERIDOL IN BODY FLUIDS

Dorota Bartusik-Aebisher, David Aebisher and Zuzanna Bober*
Faculty of Medicine, University of Rzeszów, Rzeszów, Poland

ABSTRACT

The aim of this chapter is to investigate methods for the determination of haloperidol in body fluids such as blood, urine and cerebral spinal fluid. This chapter discusses the following techniques: reaction with 1,2-naphthoquinone-4-sulphonic acid, polarography, proton (^{1}H) magnetic resonance spectroscopy, spectrophotometry, high performance liquid chromatography, and gas chromatography with mass spectrometry (GC–MS).

Keywords: fluorinated drug, Haloperidol, body fluids

---

* Corresponding Author Email: dbartusik-aebisher@ur.edu.pl.

INDICATIONS OF HALOPERIDOL

Drug concentrations in body fluids are affected by the dose, route of administration, pattern of drug use, and the dispositional kinetics (distribution, metabolism, and excretion) of the drug. Schizophrenic psychoses (acute and chronic) and other diseases listed below are often treated with haloperidol.

- manic states
- delirium
- exogenous psychosis (eg alcohol depression)
- psychomotor agitation (the so-called pharmacological straitjacket)
- organic personality disorders of old age (currently limited)
- vomiting resistant to typical treatment
- Huntington's chorea
- Sydenham's chore
- Tourette syndrome

As delirium in critically ill children is increasingly recognized, more children are treated with the antipsychotic drug haloperidol (Slooff et al. 2018). Haloperidol is metabolized to 4-(4-chlorophenyl)-4-hydroxy-piperidine and 3-(4-fluorobenzoyl)-propionic acid (Skorniakova and Lazarian 2009). 4-(4-chlorophenyl)-4-hydroxypiperidine is excreted in the urea whereas the second metabolite is not detected because it is further metabolized to 3-(4-fluorophenyl)-acetic acid (Skorniakova and Lazarian 2009). Methods for the isolation of 4-(4-chlorophenyl)-4-hydroxy-piperidine from urine, its identification, and quantitative determination have been performed using high-performance liquid chromatography (Skorniakova and Lazarian 2009). A new metabolite of Haloperidol, formed by what is equivalent to the reduction of the carbonyl group to the alcohol, has been identified in human serum, liver, and urine (Kogan et al. 1983; Pape 1981; Miyazaki et al. 1981). The detection limit for haloperidol in plasma has been found to be 5 ng/mL (El-Sayed et al. 1996). The disposition of haloperidol following administration of reduced haloperidol appears to be limited by its rate of formation and the disposition of reduced haloperidol following administration of haloperidol, is much slower than that of the parent compound (Chakraborty et al. 1989). These compounds included 4-(4-chlorophenyl)-4-hydroxypiperidine haloperidol N-oxide, reduced haloperidol, the 1,2,3,6-tetrahydropyridine analogue and its N-oxide, and the pyridinium ion from haloperidol (Fang and Gorrod 1993). Larsson and Forsman developed a high-performance liquid chromatographic method for the assay of perphenazine and its dealkylated metabolite (Larsson and Forsman 1983). Liquid chromatographic-electrospray mass spectrometric method for the determination of haloperidol and reduced haloperidol in human plasma was developed using chlorohaloperidol (Hoja et al. 1997; Nakamura et al. 1997). Haloperidol increases the effect on the central nervous system when methyldopa is used concomitantly. Fluoxetine, buspirone and quinidine increase the plasma concentration of haloperidol. Cytochrome P450 inhibitors (a group of enzymes that take part in the metabolism of medicines in the liver), especially CYP2D6, may increase haloperidol blood levels. [1-[2-fluoro-4-(1H-pyrazol-1-yl)phenyl]-5-methoxy-3-(1-phenyl-1H-pyrazol-5-yl)pyridazin-4(1H)-one] is a novel phosphodiesterase thus may produce augmented antipsychotic-like activities in combination with antipsychotics without effects on plasma prolactin levels and cataleptic responses in rodents (Suzuki et al. 2018). The parameters for haloperidol differed significantly from those previously reported, which may be an indication of a drug-drug interaction (Billups et al. 2010). Multi-walled carbon nanotubes decorated with Fe_3O_4 nanoparticles were prepared to construct a novel sensor for the determination of haloperidol by voltammetric methods (Bagheri, et al. 2014). Hence, it is important to know the concentration of antipsychotic drugs in brain tissue (Zhang et al. 2007). Haloperidol is widely used in psychiatric practice both in monotherapy and in combination with neuroleptics, phenothiazine derivatives (chlorpromasin, levomepromasin) and antidepressants (amitriptilin, imipramin) (Skorniakova et al. 2007). A LC/ESI-MS/MS method was developed and validated for simultaneous quantification of olanzapine, clozapine, ziprasidone, haloperidol, risperidone, and its active metabolite 9-hydroxyrisperidone, in rat plasma using midazolam as internal standard (Zhang et al. 2007). A rapid, sensitive and reproducible HPLC method was developed and validated for the analysis of haloperidol and its three main metabolites in human plasma (Aboul-Enein et al. 2006). Figure 1 below shows the percentage distribution of topics in the determination of haloperidol in body fluids.

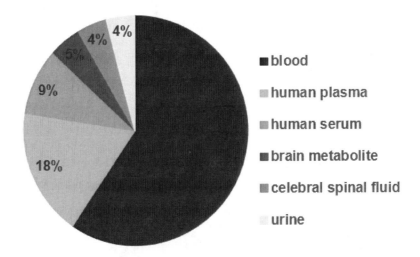

Figure 1. The statistic of determinations of haloperidol in body fluids research collected from Library of National Center for Biotechnology Information (NCBI) PubMed Data Base.

A simple and reliable gas chromatographic method with nitrogen-phosphorus detection without derivatization was developed for the detection of several psychiatric drugs in whole blood as part of systematic toxicological analyses (STA) (Sánchez de la Torre et al. 2005; Hempenius et al. 1999). Surface ionization organic mass spectrometry (SIOMS) has been performed on the fluorinated drug haloperidol using quadrupole mass spectrometry in which the thermal ion source has a rhenium oxide emitter (Fujii et al. 1996). Carbamazepine and diphenhydramine interfered with the assays of haloperidol and its metabolite, reduced haloperidol, by reversed-phase HPLC (Vatassery et al. 1993). Red blood cell (RBC) and plasma concentrations of haloperidol and reduced haloperidol were determined in nine patients who had been receiving monthly injections of haloperidol decanoate (HD) for at least 3 months. A very sensitive high performance liquid chromatography method was used to measure H and RH, which could be detected at levels as low as 0.1 ng/ml (Dysken et al. 1992). Plasma concentrations of haloperidol correlated highly with total neuroleptic activity measured by a radioreceptor assay. Compared to plasma, analysis of concentrations of haloperidol and reduced haloperidol in blood has the advantages of greater sensitivity, of using smaller volumes of blood and of avoiding the efflux of haloperidol and reduced haloperidol during separation of plasma and red cells (Eyles et al. 1992). The data indicate that reduced haloperidol is more concentrated in red blood cells than in plasma (Vatassery et al. 1990). The separation and measurement of haloperidol and hydroxy haloperidol in human plasma through high performance liquid chromatography has been developed (Pommery et al. 1990). An electrochemical HPLC method for the simultaneous determination of haloperidol and reduced haloperidol in plasma is presented with chlorohaloperidol serving as the internal standard (Eddington and Young 1988). Haloperidol and reduced haloperidol are concentrated from blood samples by liquid/liquid extraction into a hexane/isoamyl alcohol mixture, with chlorohaloperidol as the internal standard (Korpi et al. 1983). Haloperidol concentrations measured by this method correlated well with those by gas-chromatography with nitrogen-sensitive detector and by radioimmunoassay (Korpi et al. 1983). The present method can be used to study the effects of haloperidol on the central nervous system (Korpi et al. 1983). It is simple enough for use in clinical laboratories that are monitoring haloperidol concentrations in the blood of psychiatric patients (Korpi et al. 1983). A simple, highly sensitive and specific high-performance liquid chromatographic method that uses a coulometric detector for the simultaneous assay of haloperidol and reduced haloperidol in human plasma has been developed, using bromoperidol as the internal standard (Hariharan et al. 1989; Hariharan et al. 1989). A simple and highly sensitive liquid chromatographic method with electrochemical detection for the simultaneous determination of haloperidol and its metabolite reduced haloperidol in human plasma has been developed (Aravagiri et al. 1994; Aravagiri et al. 1994). A high performance liquid chromatographic method was used for the simultaneous determination of haloperidol and reduced haloperidol in human plasma, urine and rat tissue homogenates using bromperidol as an internal standard (Park et al. 1991). The formed emulsion was centrifuged and the fine droplets of solvent were floated at the top of the test tube, then it was cooled in an ice bath and the solidified solvent was transferred into a conical vial, after melt, the analysis of the extract was carried out by HPLC (Ebrahimzadeh et al. 2013). First derivative differential pulse polarography was developed and used for the quantitative analysis of chlorphenamine maleate, haloperidol, pyridoxine and their preparations. The method is simple, swift, sensitive and accurate (Liang and Zhang 1992). The electrochemical characteristics of haloperidol and related compounds, representative neuroleptics of the butyrophenone family, have been investigated as a function of pH and concentration by direct-current, alternating-current and differential-pulse polarography and cyclic voltammetry at a hanging mercury drop electrode (Vire et al., Fischer et al. 1981). Polymeric prodrugs of mPEG-PLA-haloperidol (methoxypoly (ethylene glycol)-b-poly(lactic acid)) can self-assemble into nanoscale micelle-like structures in aqueous solutions (Hans et al. 2005; Maxwell et al. 1985). The documented lower NAA in chronically treated schizophrenia patients is most likely not a simple effect of antipsychotic medications (Bustillo et al. 2006). ^{1}H-MRS studies of schizophrenia suggest an effect of the disease or of antipsychotic medications on brain N-acetyl aspartate NAA, a marker of neuronal viability (Bustillo et al. 2004). Reduced frontal N-acetylaspartate (NAA) has been repeatedly found in chronic schizophrenia and suggests neuronal loss or dysfunction (Bustillo et al. 2002). The heterogenic pharmacological response reflects the functional and physiological diversity of the therapeutic interventions, including side effects (McLoughlin et al. 2009). Numerous magnetic resonance spectroscopy has shown reductions of NAA in different brain regions in schizophrenia (Harte et al. 2005). The spectrophotometric method with an application of base line to peak technique was used for determination of active pharmaceutical ingredients at two wavelengths:

fluphenazine, pernazine, haloperidol, and promazine (Stolarczyk et al. 2009). First derivative spectrophotometry with a zero-crossing technique of measurement is used for the quantitative determination of haloperidol in the presence of methylparaben and propylparaben, which is added as antimicrobial preservatives in pharmaceuticals (Ouanês et al. 1998). Antipsychotic drugs are prescription medications used to treat psychotic disorders, such as schizophrenia, schizoaffective disorder, or psychotic (Rosado et al. 2018). Haloperidol is an effective antipsychotic drug for treatment of schizophrenia, but prolonged use can lead to debilitating side effects. This study further demonstrates the utility of murine neurochemical metabolomics as a method to advance understanding of CNS drug effects (McClay et al. 2015; da Fonseca et al. 2013). Chromatography was performed on a methylsilicone capillary column and analytes, derivatized with N-Methyl-N-(trimethylsilyl)trifluoroacetamide, were determined in the selected-ion-monitoring (SIM) mode (Pujadas et al. 2007). Detection limits are 10 μg/L for haloperidol, 20 μg/L for xylazine and 50 μg/L for azaperol; recoveries for all analytes were higher than 70% (Olmos-Carmona et al. 1999). The changes in acetylcholine release observed in this study are consistent with the known actions of some drugs or ionic conditions on striatal cholinergic neurotransmission and are evident under the condition of urethane anesthesia (Marien and Richard 1990; Wood et al. 1987). The analysis of haloperidol in human serum, utilizing gas chromatography-ammonia chemical ionization mass spectrometry has also described. (Szczepanik-van Leeuwen 1985; Hornbeck et al. 1979). A UHPLC-MS/MS method for the quantification of the studied drugs with a sample preparation based on protein precipitation was developed (Gradinaru et al. 2014).

Haloperidol is widely used and is effective against the symptoms of psychosis seen in schizophrenia (Konopaske et al. 2013; Konopaske et al. 2008). The chemical stability of haloperidol lactate injection was studied under different storage conditions by high performance thin-layer chromatography. Haloperidol lactate injection was chemically stable under all conditions studied over 15 days (Mali'n et al. 2010; Mennickent et al. 2008). A simultaneous method for the determination of haloperidol and its metabolite, reduced haloperidol, in human serum was developed by means of high-performance liquid chromatography with fluorescence detection (Mennickent et al. 2007; Greiner et al. 2007; Kishikawa et al. 2006; Yun et al. 2005).

A thin-layer chromatography densitometry method has been developed to identify and quantify haloperidol, amitriptyline, sulpiride, promazine, fluphenazine, doxepin, diazepam, trifluoperazine, clonazepam, and chlorpromazine in selected psychotropic drugs. (Maślanka et al. 2005; Igarashi et al. 2000). A high level of sensitivity may be achieved because of the absence of interferences from other drugs, metabolites, or serum components (Hoffman et al. 1994; Hayakari et al. 1987). The method was applied to an analysis of the differential activity of biogenic amines in the rat striatum, hypothalamus, and hippocampus, produced by probenecid, haloperidol and yohimbine (Kim et al. 1987). Table 1 provides a list of important studies performed on detecting haloperidol in body fluids using various analytical methods.

Table 1. List of studies performed on detecting haloperidol in body fluids using various analytical methods

Body fluid	Labeled metabolite/concentration/ sensitive/results	Detection method	References
Human plasma	Monitoring haloperidol with selected ion	Gas chromatographic mass spectrometric	Hornbeck et al. 1979
Plasma	Developed a more rapid and convenient method based on high-performance liquid chromatography (HPLC) using a reversed-phase column and a UV detector	High-performance liquid chromatographic	Miyazaki et al. 1981
Human plasma	Quantitative determination of haloperidol, the method is sensitive to at least 5 ng/ml of extracted material and is suitable for drug measurement in the therapeutic range (5-20 ng/ml) and in the toxic range (greater than 50 ng/ml).=	High-performance liquid chromatography	Kogan et al. 1983
Serum and plasma	Determination of haloperidol and reduced metabolite haloperidol, as 0.5 ng per injection is detectable	Liquid chromatography with electrochemical detection	Korpi et al. 1983

Body fluid	Labeled metabolite/concentration/ sensitive/results	Detection method	References
Brown fat	Effect of dopamine upon oxygen consumption (QO2) of brown fat, dopamine response could be blocked by haloperidol	Polarography	Maxwell et al. 1985
Human serum	Analysis of haloperidol	Gas chromatography-ammonia chemical ionization mass spectrometry	Szczepanik-van Leeuwen 1985
Plasma, serum	Extraction of haloperidol	High performance liquid chromatography	Hayakari et al. 1987
Metabolite in Rat Brain		High-performance liquid chromatography	Kim et al. 1987
Plasma	Determination of haloperidol and reduced haloperidol	High performance liquid chromatography	Eddington and Young 1988
Plasma	Interconversion between haloperidol (HAL) and reduced haloperidol (RHAL) was examined following their separate administration in low (5 mg) single oral doses to 15 young healthy male volunteers in a crossover design	Ultrasensitive HPLC method	Chakraborty et al. 1989
Plasma	Determination haloperidol and reduced haloperidol	Liquid chromatography using a coulometric detector	Hariharan et al. 1989
Human red blood cells	Determination of reduced haloperidol and haloperidol Minimum limits of quantitation for h and rh were 0.25 and 0.1 ng/ml - on 10 or 20 mg per day of oral haloperidol the rbc to plasma concentration ratios for rh and h were 2.20 +/- 0.9 (sd) and 0.81 +/- 0.26, respectively.	Liquid chromatographic	Vatassery et al. 1990
Human plasma	Determination of haloperidol and hydroxy haloperidol Limit of detection chlorohaloperidol of about 0.7 nmol/l for haloperidol and 0.67 nmol/l for hydroxy haloperidol	High performance liquid chromatography	Pommery et al. 1990
Plasma, blood, urine and tissue homogenates	Determination of haloperidol and reduced haloperidol, detection limits for haloperidol and reduced haloperidol in human plasma were both 0.5 ng/ml, and the corresponding values in human urine were both 5 ng/ml	High-performance liquid chromatography	Park et al. 1991

Table 1. (Continued)

Body fluid	Labeled metabolite/concentration/ sensitive/results	Detection method	References
Red blood cells and plasma	haloperidol decanoate pharmacokinetics	high performance liquid chromatography	Dysken et al. 1992
Human plasma and blood	determination of haloperidol and reduced haloperidol, the plasma and blood concentrations of HA were not significantly different (P greater than 0.1), accumulation of reduced haloperidol in red blood cells was also evident in the patient on oral reduced haloperidol, in whom the mean ratio of reduced haloperidol concentrations in whole blood to plasma was 3.6 +/- 1.1	high performance liquid chromatography	Eyles et al. 1992
Analyze a microsomal metabolic mixture of haloperidol	compounds included 4-(4-chlorophenyl)-4-hydroxypiperidine (CPHP), haloperidol N-oxide (HNO), reduced haloperidol (RHAL), the 1,2,3,6-tetrahydropyridine analogue and its N-oxide, and the pyridinium ion from haloperidol (HP+)	high-performance liquid chromatographic	Fang and Gorrod 1993
Plasma	determination of haloperidol and metabolite reduced haloperidol standard curve is linear over the range of 0.1 to 15 ng/ml and the lower limit of quantitation is 0.1 ng/ml for haloperidol and 0.25 ng/ml for reduced haloperidol	liquid chromatography with electrochemical detection	Aravagiri et al. 1994
Blood, serum	monitoring of haloperidol sensitivity of the chromatographic method is 0.5 ng/ml (1.3 nM) of drug in serum, and separations can be performed in a 15-min chromatographic run	high-performance liquid chromatography	Hoffman and Edkins 1994
Plasma	The detection limit for haloperidol in plasma was found to be 5 ng/mL.	high-performance liquid chromatographic	El-Sayed et al. 1996
Human serum	determination of haloperidol	surface ionization mass spectrometry and gas chromatography	Fujii et al. 1996
Human plasma	determination of haloperidol and reduced haloperidol	liquid chromatography-mass spectrometry	Hoja et al. 1997

Body fluid	Labeled metabolite/concentration/ sensitive/results	Detection method	References
Human plasma	Concentration range of haloperidol was from 0.100 to 50.0 ng ml(-1), with an inaccuracy and overall imprecision below 10% at all concentration levels	high performance liquid chromatography with turbo ion spray tandem mass spectrometric	Hempenius et al. 1999
Urine	Detection limit is 10 microg/l for haloperidol,	Gas chromatography-mass spectrometry	Olmos-Carmona and Hernández-Carrasquilla 1999
Metabolite in rat brain	Disease or of antipsychotic medications on brain N-acetyl aspartate (NAA) (haloperidol and clozapine)	High-performance liquid chromatography	Bustillo et al. 2004
Whole blood	Determination of several psychiatric drugs (mirtazapine, chlorpromazine, methotrimeprazine, clothiapine, olanzapine, clozapine, haloperidol, and thioridazine)	Gas-liquid chromatography	Sánchez de la Torre et al. 2005
Metabolite in rat brain	Determination of tissue concentrations of NAA, chronić administration of haloperidol was associated with a significant increase (+23%) in NAA in the striatum ($p<0.05$)	High-performance liquid chromatography	Harte et al. 2005
Human blood	Bioavailability and pharmacokinetics of haloperidol tablets	Liquid chromatographic electrospray mass spectrometric (LC-MS)	Yun et al. 2005
Human plasma	Rapid determination of haloperidol and its metabolites, UV detection at 230 nm was used, with the detection limits of these compounds ranging from 2 to 5 ng.	High-performance liquid chromatography	Aboul-Enein et al. 2006
Metabolite in rat brain	Effect of haloperidol on brain N-acetyl aspartate levels Factorial ANOVA of NAA concentrations revealed no significant effect of drug group ($F(1,212) = 1.5$; $p = 0.22$) or a group by brain region interaction ($F(7,212) = 1.0$; $p = 0.43$). There was a significant main effect of region ($F(7,212) = 17.8$; $p < 0.001$) with lower NAA in the striatum	Proton magnetic resonance spectroscopy	Bustillo et al. 2006

Table 1. (Continued)

Body fluid	Labeled metabolite/concentration/ sensitive/results	Detection method	References
Human serum	Determination of haloperidol and reduced haloperidol Sensitive detection of hp and rhp in human serum with a detection limit (at a signal to noise ratio of 3) of 0.22 and 0.20 ng/ml	High-performance liquid chromatography (hplc) with fluorescence detection.	Kishikawa et al. 2006
Rat brain tissue	Simultaneous determination of olanzapine, risperidone, 9-hydroxyrisperidone, clozapine, haloperidol and ziprasidone	Liquid chromatography/tandem mass spectrometry method	Zhang et al. 2007
Blood	Chemico-toxicological analysis	High-performance liquid chromatography	Skorniakova et al. 2007
Rat plasma	Simultaneous determination of olanzapine, risperidone, 9-hydroxyrisperidone, clozapine, haloperidol and ziprasidone, validated and the specificity, linearity, lower limit of quantitation (lloq), precision, accuracy, recoveries and stability were determined. Lloq was 0.1 ng/ml and correlation coefficient (r(2)) values for the linear range of 0.1-100 ng/ml were 0.997 or greater for all the analytes. The intra-day and inter-day precision and accuracy were better than 8.05%.	Liquid chromatography/tandem mass spectrometry	Zhang et al. 2007
Oral fluid	Determination of antipsychotic drugs (haloperidol, chlorpromazine and fluphenazine) Mean recovery ranged between 44.5 and 97.7% and quantification limit between 0.9 and 44.2 ng/ml oral fluid for the different analytes.	Gas chromatography-mass spectrometry	Pujadas et al. 2007
Metabolite in rat brain	Effects of a range of psychotropic drugs on rat brain metabolites (haloperidol, clozapine, olanzapine, risperidone, aripiprazole, valproate, carbamazapine and phenytoin) Antipsychotic drugs with the exception of olanzapine, consistently increased n-acetylaspartate (naa) levels in at least one brain area	Proton magnetic resonance spectroscopy	McLoughlin et al. 2009

Body fluid	Labeled metabolite/concentration/ sensitive/results	Detection method	References
Urine	Haloperidol metabolite 4-(4-chlorophenyl)-4-hydroxypipiridine	High-performance liquid chromatography	Skorniakova and Lazarian 2009
Rat plasma	Simultaneous determination of the dopamine antagonists haloperidol, its diazepane analog, and the dopamine agonist bromocriptine	Rp-hplc-dad	Billups et al. 2010
Human plasma	Determination of chlorpromazine (cpz), haloperidol, cyamemazine, quetiapine, clozapine, olanzapine (olz), and levomepromazine	Gas chromatography-tandem mass spectrometry	da Fonseca et al. 2013
Metabolite in rat brain	time-dependent effects of haloperidol on glutamine and gaba homeostasis and astrocyte activity, A 6-month haloperidol administration increased ^{13}c labeling of glutamine by [1,2-^{13}c]acetate	^{13}c magnetic resonance spectroscopy and high-performance liquid chromatography	Konopaske et al. 2013
Pharmaceutical and biological samples	Determination of haloperidol based on its adsorption on the surface of fe3o4/mwcnts.	High performance magnetite/carbon nanotube paste electrode	Bagheri et al. 2014
Human plasma	Simultaneous quantification of seven typical antipsychotic drugs (cis-chlorprothixene, flupentixol, haloperidol, levomepromazine, pipamperone, promazine and zuclopenthixol) Method was fully validated to cover large concentration ranges of 0.2-90ng/ml for haloperidol	Ultra-high performance liquid chromatography tandem mass spectrometry	Gradinaru et al. 2014
Metabolite in rat brain	Global metabolic changes in mouse brain following 3 mg/kg/day haloperidol for 28 days, Elevated n-acetyl-aspartyl-glutamate in the haloperidol-treated mice (p = 0.004),	Liquid and gas chromatography mass spectrometry	McClay et al. 2015
Human plasma and oral fluid	Determination of antipsychotic drugs (chlorpromazine, clozapine, haloperidol, olanzapine, quetiapine, cyamemazine and, levomepromazine) Limits of detection ranged from 1 to 10 ng/ml	Gas chromatography-mass spectrometry gc-ms/ms	Rosado et al. 2018

CONCLUSION

PubMed, Embase, the Cochrane Library, Elsevier, Wiley, and Ovid were searched for randomized controlled trials and prospective studies. This chapter describes the recent trends and analytical perspectives of detection of haloperidol in body fluids.

ACKNOWLEDGMENTS

Dorota Bartusik-Aebisher acknowledges support from the National Center of Science NCN (New drug delivery systems-MRI study, Grant OPUS-13 number 2017/25/B/ST4/02481).

REFERENCES

Aboul-Enein, H. Y., Ali, I., Hoenen, H. (2006). Rapid determination of haloperidol and its metabolites in human plasma by HPLC using monolithic silica column and solid-phase extraction. *Biomedical Chromatography: BMC, 20*:760-4.

Aravagiri, M., Marder, S. R., Van Putten, T., Marshall, B. D. (1994). Simultaneous determination of plasma haloperidol and its metabolite reduced haloperidol by liquid chromatography with electrochemical detection. Plasma levels in schizophrenic patients treated with oral or intramuscular depot haloperidol. *Journal of Chromatography. B, Biomedical Applications, 656*:373-81.

Bagheri, H., Afkhami, A., Panahi, Y., Khoshsafar, H., Shirzadmehr, A. (2014). Facile stripping voltammetric determination of haloperidol using a high performance magnetite/carbon nanotube paste electrode in pharmaceutical and biological samples. *Materials Science & Engineering. C, Materials for Biological Applications, 37*:264-70.

Billups, J., Jones, C., Jackson, T. L., Ablordeppey, S. Y., Spencer, S. D. (2010). Simultaneous RP-HPLC-DAD quantification of bromocriptine, haloperidol and its diazepane structural analog in rat plasma with droperidol as internal standard for application to drug-interaction pharmacokinetics. *Biomedical Chromatography*, 24:699-705.

Bustillo, J. R., Lauriello, J., Rowland, L. M., Thomson, L. M., Petropoulos, H., Hammond, R., Hart, B., Brooks, W. M. (2002). Longitudinal follow-up of neurochemical changes during the first year of antipsychotic treatment in schizophrenia patients with minimal previous medication exposure. *Schizophrenia Research*, 58:313-21.

Bustillo, J., Barrow, R., Paz, R., Tang, J., Seraji-Bozorgzad, N., Moore, G. J., Bolognani, F., Lauriello, J., Perrone-Bizzozero, N., Galloway, M. P. (2006). Long-term treatment of rats with haloperidol: lack of an effect on brain N-acetyl aspartate levels. *Neuropsychopharmacology: Official Publication of the American College of Neuropsychopharmacology*, 31:751-6.

Bustillo, J., Wolff, C., Myers-y-Gutierrez, A., Dettmer, T. S., Cooper, T. B., Allan, A., Lauriello, J., Valenzuela, C. F. (2004). Treatment of rats with antipsychotic drugs: lack of an effect on brain N-acetyl aspartate levels. *Schizophrenia Research*, 66:31-9.

Chakraborty, B. S., Hubbard, J. W., Hawes, E. M., McKay, G., Cooper, J. K., Gurnsey, T., Korchinski, E. D., Midha, K. K. (1989). Interconversion between haloperidol and reduced haloperidol in healthy volunteers. *European Journal of Clinical Pharmacology*, 37:45-8.

da Fonseca, B. M., Moreno, I. E., Barroso, M., Costa, S., Queiroz, J. A., Gallardo, E. (2013). Determination of seven selected antipsychotic drugs in human plasma using microextraction in packed sorbent and gas chromatography-tandem mass spectrometry. *Analytical and Bioanalytical Chemistry*, 405:3953-63.

Dysken, M. W., Kim, S. W., Vatassery, G., Johnson, S. B., Skare, S., Holden, L., Thomsyck, L. (1992). Haloperidol decanoate pharmacokinetics in red blood cells and plasma. *Journal of Clinical Psychopharmacology*, 12:128-32.

Ebrahimzadeh, H., Dehghani, Z., Asgharinezhad, A. A., Shekari, N., Molaei, K. (2013). Determination of haloperidol in biological samples with the aid of ultrasound-assisted emulsification microextraction followed by HPLC-DAD. *Journal of Separation Science*, *36*:1597-603.

Eddington, N. D., Young, D. (1988). Sensitive electrochemical high-performance liquid chromatography assay for the simultaneous determination of haloperidol and reduced haloperidol. *Journal of Pharmaceutical Sciences*, *77*:541-3.

El-Sayed, Y. M., Khidr, S. H., Niazy, E. M. (1996). High-Performance Liquid Chromatographic Assay for the Determination of Haloperidol in Plasma. *Journal of Liquid Chromatography & Related Technologies*, *19*:125-134.

Eyles, D. W., Whiteford, H. A., Stedman, T. J., Pond, S. M. (1992). Determination of haloperidol and reduced haloperidol in the plasma and blood of patients on depot haloperidol. *Psychopharmacology*, *106*:268-74.

Fang, J., Gorrod, J. W. (1993). High-performance liquid chromatographic method for the detection and quantitation of haloperidol and seven of its metabolites in microsomal preparations. *Journal of Chromato-graphy*, *614*(2):267-73.

Fujii, T., Hatanaka, K., Sato, G., Yasui, Y., Arimoto, H., Mitsutsuka, Y. (1996). Selective determination of haloperidol in human serum: surface ionization mass spectrometry and gas chromatography with surface ionization detection. *Journal of Chromatography. B, Biomedical Applications*, *687*:395-403.

Gradinaru, J., Vullioud, A., Eap, C. B., Ansermot, N. (2014). Quantification of typical antipsychotics in human plasma by ultra-high performance liquid chromatography tandem mass spectrometry for therapeutic drug monitoring. *Journal of Pharmaceutical and Biomedical Analysis*, *88*:36-44.

Greiner, C., Hiemke, C., Bader, W., Haen, E. (2007). Determination of citalopram and escitalopram together with their active main metabolites desmethyl(es-)citalopram in human serum by column-switching high performance liquid chromatography (HPLC) and spectrophotometric detection. *Journal of Chromatography. B, Analytical Technologies in the Biomedical and Life Sciences*, *848*:391-4.

Hans, M., Shimoni, K., Danino, D., Siegel, S. J., Lowman, A. (2005). Synthesis and characterization of mPEG-PLA prodrug micelles. *Biomacromolecules*, *6*:2708-17.

Hariharan, M., Kindt, E. K., VanNoord, T., Tandon, R. (1989). An improved sensitive assay for simultaneous determination of plasma haloperidol and reduced haloperidol levels by liquid chromatography using a coulometric detector. *Therapeutic Drug Monitoring*, *11*:701-7.

Harte, M. K., Bachus, S. B., Reynolds, G. P. (2005). Increased N-acetylaspartate in rat striatum following long-term administration of haloperidol. *Schizophrenia Research*, *75*:303-8.

Hayakari, M., Hashimoto, Y., Kita, T., Murakami, S. (1987). A rapid and simplified extraction of haloperidol from plasma or serum with bond elut C18 cartridge for analysis by high performance liquid chromatography. *Forensic Science International*, *35*:73-81.

Hempenius, J., Steenvoorden, R. J., Lagerwerf, F. M., Wieling, J., Jonkman, J. H. (1999). 'High throughput' solid-phase extraction technology and turbo ionspray LC-MS-MS applied to the determination of haloperidol in human plasma. *Journal of Pharmaceutical and biomedical Analysis*, *20*:889-98.

Hoffman, D. W., Edkins, R. D. (1994). Solid-phase extraction and high-performance liquid chromatography for therapeutic monitoring of haloperidol levels. *Therapeutic Drug Monitoring*, *16*:504-8.

Hoja, H., Marquet, P., Verneuil, B., Lotfi, H., Dupuy, J. L., Pénicaut, B., Lachâtre, G. (1997). Determination of haloperidol and its reduced metabolite in human plasma by liquid chromatography-mass spectrometry with electrospray ionization. *Journal of Chromatography. B, Biomedical Sciences and Applications*, *688*:275-80.

Hornbeck, C. L., Griffiths, J. C., Neborsky, R. J., Faulkner, M. A. (1979). A gas chromatographic mass spectrometric chemical ionization assay for haloperidol with selected ion monitoring. *Biomedical Mass Spectrometry*, 6:427-30.

Igarashi, K., Sugiyama, Y., Kasuya, F., Inoue, H., Matoba, R., Castagnoli, N. Analysis of citrulline in rat brain tissue after perfusion with haloperidol by liquid chromatography-mass spectrometry (2000). *Journal of chromatography. B, Biomedical Sciences and Applications*, 746:33-40.

Kim, C., Speisky, M. B., Kharouba, S. N. (1987). Rapid and sensitive method for measuring norepinephrine, dopamine, 5-hydroxytryptamine and their major metabolites in rat brain by high-performance liquid chromatography. Differential effect of probenecid, haloperidol and yohimbine on the concentrations of biogenic amines and metabolites in various regions of rat brain. *Journal of Chromatography*, 386:25-35.

Kishikawa, N., Hamachi, C., Imamura, Y., Ohba, Y., Nakashima, K., Tagawa, Y., Kuroda, N. (2006). Determination of haloperidol and reduced haloperidol in human serum by liquid chromatography after fluorescence labeling based on the Suzuki coupling reaction. *Analytical and Bioanalytical Chemistry*, 386:719-24.

Kogan, M. J., Pierson, D., Verebey, K. (1983). Quantitative determination of haloperidol in human plasma by high-performance liquid chromatography. *Therapeutic Drug Monitoring*, 5:485-9.

Konopaske, G. T., Bolo, N. R., Basu, A. C., Renshaw, P. F., Coyle, J. T. (2013). Time-dependent effects of haloperidol on glutamine and GABA homeostasis and astrocyte activity in the rat brain. *Psychopharmacology*, 230:57-67.

Korpi, E. R., Phelps, B. H., Granger, H., Chang, W. H., Linnoila, M., Meek, J. L., Wyatt, R. J. (1983). Simultaneous determination of haloperidol and its reduced metabolite in serum and plasma by isocratic liquid chromatography with electrochemical detection. *Clinical Chemistry*, 29:624-8.

Larsson, M., Forsman, A. (1983). A high-performance liquid chromatographic method for the assay of perphenazine and its dealkylated metabolite in serum after therapeutic doses. *Therapeutic Drug Monitoring*, 5:225-8.

Liang, Y. A., Zhang, T. M. (1992). Studies on first derivative differential pulse polarography and its applications. *Acta Pharmaceutica Sinica*, *27*:135-8.

Mali'n, T. J., Weidolf, L., Castagnoli, N. Jr., Jurva, U. (2010). P450-catalyzed vs. electrochemical oxidation of haloperidol studied by ultra-performance liquid chromatography/electrospray ionization mass spectrometry. *Rapid Communications in Mass Spectrometry: RCM*, *24*:1231-40.

Marien, M. R., Richard, J. W. (1990). Drug effects on the release of endogenous acetylcholine *in vivo*: measurement by intracerebral dialysis and gas chromatography-mass spectrometry. *Journal of Neurochemistry*, *54*:2016-23.

Maślanka, A., Krzek, J. (2005). Densitometric high performance thin-layer chromatography identification and quantitative analysis of psychotropic drugs. *Journal of AOAC International*, *88*:70-9.

Maxwell, G., Crompton, S., Smyth, C. (1985). The effect of dopamine upon oxidative metabolism of brown fat adipocytes. *European Journal of Pharmacology*, *116*:293-7.

McClay, J. L., Vunck, S. A., Batman, A. M., Crowley, J. J., Vann, R. E., Beardsley, P. M., van den Oord, E. J. (2015). Neurochemical Metabolomics Reveals Disruption to Sphingolipid Metabolism Following Chronic Haloperidol Administration. *Journal of Neuroimmune Pharmacology: the Official Journal of the Society on NeuroImmune Pharmacology*, *10*:425-34.

McLoughlin, G. A., Ma, D., Tsang, T. M., Jones, D. N., Cilia, J., Hill, M. D., Robbins, M. J., Benzel, I. M., Maycox, P. R., Holmes, E., Bahn, S. (2009). Analyzing the effects of psychotropic drugs on metabolite profiles in rat brain using 1H NMR spectroscopy. *Journal of Proteome Research*, *8*:1943-52.

Mennickent, S., Pino, L., Vega, M., de Diego, M. (2008). Chemical stability of haloperidol injection by high performance thin-layer chromatography. *Journal of Separation Science*, *31*:201-6.

Mennickent, S., Pino, L., Vega, M., Godoy, C. G., de Diego, M. (2007). Quantitative determination of haloperidol in tablets by high performance thin-layer chromatography. *Journal of Separation Science, 30:*772-7.

Miyazaki, K., Arita, T., Oka, I., Koyama, T., Yamashita, I. (1981). High-performance liquid chromatographic determination of haloperidol in plasma. *Journal of Chromatography B: Biomedical Sciences and Applications, 223:*449-453.

Nakamura, J., Uchimura, N., Yamada, S., Nakazawa, Y. (1997). Does plasma free-3-methoxy-4-hydroxyphenyl(ethylene)glycol increase in the delirious state? A comparison of the effects of mianserin and haloperidol on delirium. *International Clinical Psychopharmacology, 12:*147-52.

Olmos-Carmona, M. L., Hernández-Carrasquilla, M. (1999). Gas chromatographic-mass spectrometric analysis of veterinary tranquillizers in urine: evaluation of method performance. *Journal of Chromatography. B, Biomedical Sciences and Applications, 734:*113-20.

Ouanês, S., Kallel, M., Trabelsi, H., Safta, F., Bouzouita, K. (1998). Zero-crossing derivative spectrophotometry for the determination of haloperidol in presence of parabens. *Journal of Pharmaceutical and Biomedical Analysis, 17:*361-4.

Pape, B. E. Isolation and Identification of a Metabolite of haloperidol. (1981). *Journal of Analytical Toxicology, 5:*113–117.

Park, K. H., Lee, M. H., Lee, M. G. (1991). Simultaneous determination of haloperidol and its metabolite, reduced haloperidol, in plasma, blood, urine and tissue homogenates by high-performance liquid chromatography. *Journal of Chromatography, 572:*259-67.

Pommery, J., Foulon, O., Morineau, G., Lhermitte, M., Levron, J. C., Erb, F. (1990). Determination of haloperidol and hydroxy haloperidol in human plasma by high performance liquid chromatography. *Annales de Biologie Clinique, 48:*455-8.

Pujadas, M., Pichini, S., Civit, E., Santamariña, E., Perez, K., de la Torre, R. (2007). A simple and reliable procedure for the determination of psychoactive drugs in oral fluid by gas chromatography-mass spectrometry. *Journal of Pharmaceutical and Biomedical Analysis, 44*:594-601.

Rosado, T., Oppolzer, D., Cruz, B., Barroso, M., Varela, S., Oliveira, V., Leitão, C., Gallardo, E. (2018). Development and validation of GC/MS/MS method for simultaneous quantitation of several antipsychotics in human plasma and oral fluid. *Rapid Communications in Mass Spectrometry: RCM*, doi: 10.1002/rcm.8087.

Sánchez de la Torre, C., Martínez, M. A., Almarza, E. (2005). Determination of several psychiatric drugs in whole blood using capillary gas-liquid chromatography with nitrogen phosphorus detection: comparison of two solid phase extraction procedures. *Forensic Science International, 155*(2-3):193-204.

Skorniakova, A. B., Lazarian, D. S. (2009). Chemical toxicological analysis of haloperidol metabolite 4-(4-chlorophenyl)-4-hydroxy-pipiridine in urine by high-performance liquid chromatography. *Sudebno-Meditsinskaia Ekspertiza, 52*:45-8.

Skorniakova, A. B., Lazarian, D. S., Tsybulina, M. G. (2007). Chemico-toxicological analysis of haloperidol in blood with high-performance liquid chromatography in combined poisoning. *Sudebno-Meditsinskaia Ekspertiza, 50*:33-5.

Slooff, V. D., van den Dungen, D. K., van Beusekom, B. S., Jessurun, N., Ista, E., Tibboel, D., de Wildt, S. N. (2018). Monitoring Haloperidol Plasma Concentration and Associated Adverse Events in Critically Ill Children With Delirium: First Results of a Clinical Protocol Aimed to Monitor Efficacy and Safety. *Pediatric Critical Care Medicine: a Journal of the Society of Critical Care Medicine and the World Federation of Pediatric Intensive and Critical Care Societies, 19*:112-9.

Stolarczyk, M., Apola, A., Krzek, J., Sajdak, A. (2009). Validation of derivative spectrophotometry method for determination of active ingredients from neuroleptics in pharmaceutical preparations. *Acta Poloniae Pharmaceutica, 66*:351-6.

Suzuki, K., Harada, A., Suzuki, H., Capuani, C., Ugolini, A., Corsi, M., Kimura, H. (2018). Combined treatment with a selective PDE10A inhibitor TAK-063 and either haloperidol or olanzapine at subeffective doses produces potent antipsychotic-like effects without affecting plasma prolactin levels and cataleptic responses in rodents. *Pharmacology Research & Perspectives*, 6.

Szczepanik-van Leeuwen, P. A. (1985). Improved gas chromatographic-mass spectrometric assay for haloperidol utilizing ammonia chemical ionization and selected-ion monitoring. *Journal of Chromatography*, *339*:321-30.

Trabelsi, H., Bouabdallah, S., Bouzouita, K., Safta, F. (2002). Determination and degradation study of haloperidol by high performance liquid chromatography. *Journal of Pharmaceutical and Biomedical Analysis*, *29*:649-57.

Vatassery, G. T., Herzan, L. A., Dysken, M. W. (1990). Liquid chromatographic determination of reduced haloperidol and haloperidol concentrations in packed red blood cells from humans. *Journal of Analytical Toxicology*, *14*:25-8.

Vatassery, G. T., Holden, L. A., Dysken, M. W. (1993). Resolution of the interference from carbamazepine and diphenhydramine during reversed-phase liquid chromatographic determination of haloperidol and reduced haloperidol. *Journal of Analytical Toxicology*, *17*:304-6.

Vire, J. C., Fischer, M., Patriarche, G. J., Christian, G. D. (1981). Electrochemical behaviour of some neuroleptics: Haloperidol and its derivatives. *Talanta*, *28*:313-7.

Wood, P. L., Kim, H. S., Altar, C. A. (1987). *In vivo* assessment of dopamine and norepinephrine release in rat neocortex: gas chromatography-mass spectrometry measurement of 3-methoxytyramine and normetanephrine. *Journal of Neurochemistry*, *48*:574-9.

Yun, M. H., Kwon, J. T., Kwon, K. I. (2005). Pharmacokinetics and bioequivalence of haloperidol tablet by liquid chromatographic mass spectrometry with electrospray ionization. *Archives of Pharmacal Research*, *28*:488-92.

Zhang, G., Terry, A. V. Jr., Bartlett, M. G. (2007). Liquid chromatography/tandem mass spectrometry method for the simultaneous determination of olanzapine, risperidone, 9-hydroxyrisperidone, clozapine, haloperidol and ziprasidone in rat plasma. *Rapid Communications in Mass Spectrometry: RCM, 21*:920-8.

Zhang, G., Terry, A. V. Jr., Bartlett, M. G. (2007). Sensitive liquid chromatography/tandem mass spectrometry method for the simultaneous determination of olanzapine, risperidone, 9-hydroxyrisperidone, clozapine, haloperidol and ziprasidone in rat brain tissue. *Journal of Chromatography. B, Analytical Technologies in the Biomedical and Life Sciences, 858*:276-81.

In: The Pharmacological Guide to Haloperidol   ISBN: 978-1-53614-700-1
Editor: Amor Harland   © 2019 Nova Science Publishers, Inc.

Chapter 3

MEDICAL APPLICATIONS OF HALOPERIDOL DERIVATIVES

David Aebisher, Dorota Bartusik-Aebisher and Łukasz Ożóg*

Faculty of Medicine, University of Rzeszów, Rzeszów, Poland

ABSTRACT

Haloperidol and its derivatives are mainly used as antipsychotics, although other potential medical uses have been described in the literature. In this chapter, a description of haloperidol derivatives and their applications as antimicrobial agents, vasodilators, and calcium channel blockers are discussed. Additionally, haloperidol derivatives that have potential applications in improving cardiac function and reducing oxidative stress will also be addressed.

Keywords: haloperidol, antipsychotic, oxidative stress.

* Corresponding Author Email: daebisher@ur.edu.pl.

Haloperidol is an antipsychotic drug with known antimicrobial properties that contains a fluorophenyl and chlorophenyl residue on a piperidine skeleton (Holbrook et al. 2017; Stylianou et al. 2014). Haloperidol is an antipsychotic agent and acts as dopamine D2 receptor antagonist (Lencesova et al. 2017; Kim et al. 2017). Antipsychotic effects occur with negligible anticholinergic activity, probably due to its strong affinity for the D2 receptor. Haloperidol also has a strong sedative effect and is a moderate antispastic agent with depressant action. The poor anticholinergic action of haloperidol on the one hand protects against delirium disorders, but is also responsible for the depressive effect.

Indications of Haloperidol:

- Schizophrenia and schizoaffective psychoses
- Manic states
- Conditions of aggression and psychomotor agitation
- Attitudes towards violence in patients with brain dysfunction or in the mentally impaired

Haloperidol is one of the strongest neuroleptic drugs available and is about 50 times stronger than chlorpromazine. Related compounds in which chlorine is replaced by a trifluoromethyl group (for example trifluperidol) or bromine instead of chlorine in bromoperidol are even more potent. Haloperidol reduces the psychomotor drive and anxiety. It also acts as an antiemetic agent effectively inhibiting nausea and hiccups. Haloperidol was investigated as a potential agent to improve *M. tuberculosis* efflux-inhibition (Machado et al. 2016; Seki et al. 2013) and its use as both a vasodilator and calcium channel blocker has been intensively studied (Zhang et al. 2013; Reiriz et al. 1994; Neumaier and Chavkin 1989; Lau and Gnegy 1982). Derivatives of haloperidol developed by Chen and coworkers were found to be novel calcium antagonists with stronger vasodilation effects with less cardiac side effects than the parent compound (Chen et al. 2015; Park et al. 2015; Shi et al. 2001). Several haloperidol derivatives with a piperidine scaffold were screened for vasodilatory activity (Chen et al. 2011). Both N-n-butyl haloperidol iodide (Huang et al. 2007) and N-4-Tert-Butyl benzyl haloperidol chloride (Xiao et al. 2011; Chen et al. 2009; Tarabová et al. 2009; Kim et al. 2006) have been reported to act as calcium antagonists. Haloperidol may serve as a potential agent in alleviating the neurotoxic effects of beta-amyloid peptide (Palotás et al. 2004). Haloperidol is a classical neuroleptic drug that can lead to abnormal motor activity such as tardive dyskinesia following repeated administration (Yang et al. 2011; Bishnoi et al. 2008; Lee et al. 2007; Belforte et al. 2001; Nalepa et al. 1999; Esteve et al. 1995). N-n-butyl haloperidol iodide is a novel quaternary ammonium salt derivative of haloperidol that has been found to antagonize myocardial ischemia (Huang et al. 2012; Zhang et al. 2012; Jomphe et al. 2003; Guenther et al. 1994). The effect of verapamil, nifedipine, diltiazem, cinnarizine, and fendilin on haloperidol-induced catalepsy have been studied (Kozlovskiĭ et al. 1996). Cellular calcium (Ca^{2+}) regulation which is effected by haloperidol derivatives has been implicated as an important mechanism in certain diseases such as bipolar affective disorder (Biała 2000; Brent et al. 1996; Sczekan and Strumwasser 1996).

Low dose haloperidol (1-2 mg every 2 to 4 hours) has been used to treat agitated cardiac patients (Henderson et al. 1991; Tesar et al. 1985). Intravenously delivered haloperidol is the drug of choice for controlling severe delirium in agitated cardiac patients. Prior reports have warned that high-dose intravenous haloperidol can cause torsades de pointes (abnormal heart rhythm) in some patients treated (Di Salvo et al. 1995; Metzger et al. 1993). Haloperidol and lorazepam are commonly used to sedate ethanol intoxicated patients in emergency rooms and studies have been conducted to explore the role of ethanol in altering the potency of haloperidol and lorazepam with respect to cardiac conduction and contraction (Medlin et al. 1996).

Haloperidol is also used as a neuroleptic drug for treatment of various psychoses and deliria. Haloperidol binds to sigma receptors that are coupled with inositol 1,4,5-trisphosphate (IP3) receptors (Stracina et al. 2015; Novakova et al. 2010). Haloperidol has been reported to induce polymorphic ventricular arrhythmias (Satoh et al. 2000). A comparative study of the cardiovascular effects of aripiprazole and haloperidol using a halothane-anesthetized canine model with monophasic action potential monitoring was reported (Sugiyama et al. 2001). Haloperidol administration (0.02 mg/kg/min intravenously) was found to induce a significant, rate-dependent slowing of intraventricular conduction (Mörtl et al. 2003). Sufficient restoration of original heart beat profiles following haloperidol treatment were reported after drug removal (Liu et al. 2017). Haloperidol also binds to the sigma-1 receptor (σ1R) and inhibits it irreversibly (Shinoda et al. 2016; Howland 2014). Autopsy data suggests that orally administered haloperidol is not associated with an increased risk of sudden cardiac death in psychiatric inpatients with dementia (Ifteni et al. 2015; Atalan et al. 2013). No significant differences in QTc (corrected QT interval) prolongation, adverse events, or need for repeated sedation was found between haloperidol and droperidol in a prehospital setting (Macht et al. 2014; Scharfetter and Fischer 2014). Treatment with the neuroleptic agent haloperidol is sometimes associated with serious cardiac arrhythmias (Lu et al. 2016; Armahizer et al. 2013; Mörtl et al. 2003) and pharmacovigilance is needed to ensure the safe and effective use of this class of medicine (Vandael et al. 2016; Meyer-Massetti et al. 2011; Gao et al. 2010; Warnier et al. 2015; Wang and Wang 2015; Muzyk et al. 2012; Meyer-Massetti et al. 2010). Haloperidol, in contrast to citalopram and escitalopram, can cause a significant increase in dispersion of repolarization in heart muscle (Frommeyer et al. 2016; Raghu et al. 2009). This effect of haloperidol reflects an alteration of endogenous electrical properties of the constituent neurons, rather than receptor antagonism (Akers et al. 2004; Berlind 2001) and reports suggest that low-dose thioridazine and haloperidol have similar cardiac safety (Hennessy et al. 2004). The cardiac effects of haloperidol as a sigma receptor ligand have been studied extensively in humans as well as in various animal models, primarily after acute administration (Fialova et al. 2009). Despite these reports, intravenous haloperidol has a reputation for safe and effective sedation of patients and has been found to be free of many of the dangerous anticholinergic and cardiac side effects of lower-potency neuroleptics (Iwahashi 1996; Metzger and Friedman 1993; Fulop et al. 1987). Haloperidol is widely prescribed for schizophrenia and other affective disorders but has severe side effects such as tardive dyskinesia (Sagara 1998). Haloperidol is cytotoxic to cells of different origin in high doses (Behl et al. 1996; Post et al. 1998). Haloperidol has been hypothesized to potentiate increases in oxidative stress and free radical-mediated levels of toxic metabolites in rat striatum while simultaneously upregulating dopamine (DA) D2 receptors leading to presumed DA super sensitivity. Results of these experiments show that haloperidol induced VCMs (vacuous chewing movements) in rats results from an increase in oxidative cellular events and may not be related to increases in striatal DA D(2) receptors (Rogoza et al. 2004). Tardive dyskinesia is a complex hyperkinetic syndrome consisting of both choreiform and athetoid movements which can persist for months or years after haloperidol withdrawal (Thaakur and Himabindhu 2009). There is evidence that reactive oxygen species are involved in the pathophysiology of psychiatric disorders such as schizophrenia (Heiser et al. 2010). Haloperidol is a classic antipsychotic drug and is known to induce oxidative stress due to increased turnover of dopamine (El-Awdan et al. 2015). Interestingly, there is also evidence that reactive oxygen species are involved in the pathophysiology of psychiatric disorders such as schizophrenia (Heiser et al. 2010). Haloperidol and its metabolites have been found to be both neurotoxic and cardiotoxic (Raudenska et al. 2013). The findings of the present study suggest the involvement of striatal free radicals in the development of behavioral supersensitivity, and the use of free radical trapping agents as possible options for the treatment of extrapyramidal side effects in humans (Abdel-Sattar et al. 2014; Bošković et al. 2013; Daya et al. 2011). Studies describing haloperidol in various fields by percent between 1972 and 2017 collected from the Library of the National Center for Biotechnology Information (NCBI) PubMed Data Base are shown in Figure 1.

Haloperidol 1972-2017

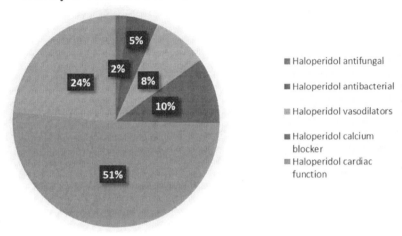

Figure 1. Studies of haloperidol between 1972 and 2017 arranged by application and percent resulting from publications collected from Library of National Center for Biotechnology Information (NCBI) PubMed Data Base.

The antioxidant activity of superoxide dismutase, catalase, glutathione peroxidase, glutathione reductase, malondialdehyde, protein carbonyls, nitrite, nitrate, glutathione, dopamine, noradrenaline, adrenaline, and serotonin were measured in 52 outpatients with a DSM-IV diagnosis of schizophrenia that were treated with haloperidol decanoate (Bošković et al. 2013; Zhang et al. 2012). Studies conducted by Andreazza and coworkers suggest that haloperidol may induce oxidative stress in the brain (Andreazza et al. 2015; Gawlik-Kotelnicka et al. 2015). A recent report indicates that lithium possesses neuroprotective properties that may be partly due to an antioxidative effect and that the combination of lithium and haloperidol generates increased oxidative stress (Gawlik-Kotelnicka et al. 2016). Haloperidol is the most widely used antipsychotic drug in the treatment of psychiatric disorders (Benvegnú et al. 2012). Further evidence for toxicity was found from a study that demonstrated that haloperidol administration causes significant oxidative stress in guinea pigs (Gumulec et al. 2013; Nade et al. 2010). Reactive oxygen species induce cytoskeletal collapse and excessive phosphorylation of tau, a microtubule-associated protein that plays a key role in microtubule stabilization, growth cone development, and neurite formation, which are cytoskeletal phenotypes that participate in neurodevelopment (Benítez-King et al. 2010). Haloperidol causes extrapyramidal symptoms (Abdel-Salam et al. 2012; Shivakumar and Ravindranath 1992). Haloperidol is an antipsychotic drug that exerts its antipsychotic effects by inhibiting dopaminergic neurons. Although the exact pathophysiology of haloperidol extrapyramidal symptoms are not known, the role of reactive oxygen species in inducing oxidative stress has been proposed as one of the mechanisms of prolonged haloperidol-induced neurotoxicity (Perera et al. 2011; Thaakur and Jyothi 2007).

CONCLUSION

Haloperidol and its derivatives are mainly used as antipsychotics, however, other potential medical uses have been described in the literature. In this chapter, a description of haloperidol derivatives and their applications as antifungal and antibacterial agents, vasodilators, and calcium channel blockers are discussed. Additionally, haloperidol derivatives that have potential applications in improving cardiac function and reducing oxidative stress were addressed as well as the neurotoxic and cardiotoxic side effects of the parent drug haloperidol.

ACKNOWLEDGMENTS

Dorota Bartusik-Aebisher acknowledges support from the National Center of Science NCN (New drug delivery systems-MRI study, Grant OPUS-13 number 2017/25/B/ST4/02481)

REFERENCES

Abdel-Salam, O. M., El-Sayed El-Shamarka, M., Salem, N. A. & El-Din M Gaafar, A. (2012). Effects of Cannabis sativa extract on haloperidol-induced catalepsy and oxidative stress in the mice. *Experimental and Clinical Sciences Journal, 11*, 45-58.

Abdel-Sattar, E. A., Mouneir, S. M., Asaad, G. F. & Abdallah, H. M. (2014). Protective effect of *Calligonum comosum* on haloperidol-induced oxidative stress in rat. *Toxicology and Industrial Health, 30*(2), 147-53.

Akers, W. S., Flynn, J. D., Davis, G. A., Green, A. E., Winstead, P. S. & Strobel, G. (2004). Prolonged cardiac repolarization after tacrolimus and haloperidol administration in the critically ill patient. *Pharmacotherapy, 24*(3), 404-8.

Andreazza, A. C., Barakauskas, V. E., Fazeli, S., Feresten, A., Shao, L., Wei, V., Wu, C. H., Barr, A. M. & Beasley, C. L. (2015). Effects of haloperidol and clozapine administration on oxidative stress in rat brain, liver and serum. *Neuroscience Letters, 591*, 36-40.

Armahizer, M. J., Seybert, A. L., Smithburger, P. L. & Kane-Gill, S. L. (2013). Drug-drug interactions contributing to QT prolongation in cardiac intensive care units. *Journal of Critical Care, 28*(3), 243-9.

Atalan, N., Efe Sevim, M., Akgün, S., Fazlıoğulları, O. & Başaran, C. (2013). Morphine is a reasonable alternative to haloperidol in the treatment of postoperative hyperactive-type delirium after cardiac surgery. *Journal of Cardiothoracic and Vascular Anesthesia, 27*(5), 933-8.

Behl, C., Lezoualc'h, F., Widmann, M., Rupprecht, R. & Holsboer, F. (1996). Oxidative stress-resistant cells are protected against haloperidol toxicity. *Brain Research, 717*(1-2), 193-5.

Belforte, J. E., Magariños-Azcone, C., Armando, I., Buño, W. & Pazo, J. H. (2001). Pharmacological involvement of the calcium channel blocker flunarizine in dopamine transmission at the striatum. *Parkinsonism and Related Disorders, 8*(1), 33-40.

Benítez-King, G., Ortíz-López, L., Jiménez-Rubio, G. & Ramírez-Rodríguez, G. (2010). Haloperidol causes cytoskeletal collapse in N1E-115 cells through tau hyperphosphorylation induced by oxidative stress: Implications for neurodevelopment. *European Journal of Pharmacology*, *644*(1-3), 24-31.

Benvegnú, D. M., Barcelos, R. C., Boufleur, N., Pase, C. S., Reckziegel, P., Flores, F. C., Ourique, A. F., Nora, M. D., da Silva Cde, B., Beck, R. C. & Bürger, M. E. (2012). Haloperidol-loaded polysorbate-coated polymeric nanocapsules decrease its adverse motor side effects and oxidative stress markers in rats. *Neurochemistry International*, *61*(5), 623-31.

Berlind, A. (2001). Effects of haloperidol and phentolamine on the crustacean cardiac ganglion. *Comparative Biochemistry and Physiology. Toxicology and Pharmacology: CBP*, *130*(1), 85-95.

Biała, G. (2000). Haloperidol-induced catalepsy is influenced by calcium channel antagonists. *Acta Poloniae Pharmaceutica*, *57*(3), 233-7.

Bishnoi, M., Chopra, K. & Kulkarni, S. K. (2008). Protective effect of L-type calcium channel blockers against haloperidol-induced orofacial dyskinesia: a behavioural, biochemical and neurochemical study. *Neurochemical Research*, *33*(9), 1869-80.

Bošković, M., Grabnar, I., Terzič, T., Kores Plesničar, B. & Vovk, T. (2013). Oxidative stress in schizophrenia patients treated with long-acting haloperidol decanoate. *Psychiatry Research*, *210*(3), 761-8.

Brent, P. J., Pang, G., Little, G., Dosen, P. J. & Van Helden, D. F. (1996). The sigma receptor ligand, reduced haloperidol, induces apoptosis and increases intracellular-free calcium levels [Ca2+]i in colon and mammary adenocarcinoma cells. *Biochemical and Biophysical Research Communications*, *219*(1), 219-26.

Chen, Y. C., Zhu, W., Zhong, S. P., Zheng, F. C., Gao, F. F., Zhang, Y. M., Xu, H., Zheng, Y. S. & Shi, G. G. (2015). Characterization and bioactivity of novel calcium antagonists- N-methoxy-benzyl haloperidol quaternary ammonium salt. *Oncotarget*, *6*(41), 43759-69.

Chen, Y., Zheng, J., Zhang, Y., Wang, J., Liu, Q., Huang, Z., Gao, F., Zhou, Y. & Shi, G. (2009). N-4-tert-butyl benzyl haloperidol chloride suppresses Ca2+-dependent Egr-1 expression and subsequently inhibits vascular smooth muscle cell proliferation induced by angiotensin II. *Cellular Physiology and Biochemistry: International Journal of Experimental Cellular Physiology, Biochemistry, and Pharmacology, 23*(4-6), 295-304.

Chen, Y., Zheng, J., Zheng, F., Wang, J., Zhang, Y., Gao, F., Huang, Z. & Shi, G. (2011). Design, synthesis, and pharmacological evaluation of haloperidol derivatives as novel potent calcium channel blockers with vasodilator activity. *Public Library of Science One PLoS 1, 6*(11), e27673.

Daya, R. P., Tan, M. L., Sookram, C. D., Skoblenick, K. & Mishra, R. K. (2011). Alpha-phenyl-N-tert-butylnitrone prevents oxidative stress in a haloperidol-induced animal model of tardive dyskinesia: investigating the behavioural and biochemical changes. *Brain Research, 1412*, 28-36.

Di Salvo, T. G. & O'Gara, P. T. (1995). Torsade de pointes caused by high-dose intravenous haloperidol in cardiac patients. *Clinical Cardiology, 18*(5), 285-90.

El-Awdan, S. A., Abdel Jaleel, G. A. & Saleh, D. O. (2015). Alleviation of haloperidol induced oxidative stress in rats: Effects of sucrose vs grape seed extract, *Bulletin of Faculty of Pharmacy,* Cairo University, *53*(1), 29-35.

Esteve, L., Haby, C., Rodeau, J. L., Humblot, N., Aunis, D. & Zwiller, J. (1995). Induction of c-fos, jun B and egr-1 expression by haloperidol in PC12 cells: involvement of calcium. *Neuropharmacology, 34*(4), 439-48.

Fialova, K., Krizanova, O., Jarkovsky, J. & Novakova, M. (2009). Apparent desensitization of the effects of sigma receptor ligand haloperidol in isolated rat and guinea pig hearts after chronic treatment. *Canadian Journal of Physiology and Pharmacology, 87*(12), 1019-27.

Frommeyer, G., Brücher, B., von der Ahe, H., Kaese, S., Dechering, D. G., Kochhäuser, S., Bogossian, H., Milberg, P. & Eckardt, L. (2016). Low proarrhythmic potential of citalopram and escitalopram in contrast to haloperidol in an experimental whole-heart model. *European Journal of Pharmacology*, *788*, 192-9.

Fulop, G., Phillips, R. A., Shapiro, A. K., Gomes, J. A., Shapiro, E. & Nordlie, J. W. (1987). ECG changes during haloperidol and pimozide treatment of Tourette's disorder. *The American Journal of Psychiatry*, *144*(5), 673-5.

Gao, F. F., Hao, S. Y., Huang, Z. Q., Zhang, Y. M., Zhou, Y. Q., Chen, Y. C., Liu, X. P. & Shi, G. G. (2010). Cardiac electrophysiological and antiarrhythmic effects of N-n-butyl haloperidol iodide. *Cellular Physiology and Biochemistry: International Journal of Experimental Cellular Physiology, Biochemistry, and Pharmacology*, *25*(4-5), 433-42.

Gawlik-Kotelnicka, O., Mielicki, W., Rabe-Jabłońska, J., Lazarek, J. & Strzelecki, D. (2016). Impact of lithium alone or in combination with haloperidol on oxidative stress parameters and cell viability in SH-SY5Y cell culture. *Acta Neuropsychiatrica*, *28*(1), 38-44.

Gawlik-Kotelnicka, O., Mielicki, W., Rabe-Jabłońska, J. & Strzelecki, D. (2015). Impact of lithium alone or in combination with haloperidol on selected oxidative stress parameters in human plasma *in vitro. Redox Report: Communications in Free Radical Research*, *21*(1), 45-9.

Guenther, E., Wilsch, V. & Zrenner, E. (1994). Inhibitory action of haloperidol, spiperone and SCH23390 on calcium currents in rat retinal ganglion cells. *Neuroreport*, *5*(11), 1373-6.

Gumulec, J., Raudenska, M., Hlavna, M., Stracina, T., Sztalmachova, M., Tanhauserova, V., Pacal, L., Ruttkay-Nedecky, B., Sochor, J., Zitka, O., Babula, P., Adam, V., Kizek, R., Novakova, M. & Masarik, M. (2013). Determination of oxidative stress and activities of antioxidant enzymes in guinea pigs treated with haloperidol. *Experimental and Therapeutic Medicine*, *5*(2), 479-84.

Heiser, P., Sommer, O., Schmidt, A. J., Clement, H. W., Hoinkes, A., Hopt, U. T., Schulz, E., Krieg, J. C. & Dobschütz, E. (2010). Effects of antipsychotics and vitamin C on the formation of reactive oxygen species. *Journal of Psychopharmacology/British Association for Psychopharmacology*, *24*(10), 1499-504.

Henderson, R. A., Lane, S. & Henry, J. A. (1991). Life-threatening ventricular arrhythmia (torsades de pointes) after haloperidol overdose. *Human and Experimental Toxicology*, *10*(1), 59-62.

Hennessy, S., Bilker, W. B., Knauss, J. S., Kimmel, S. E., Margolis, D. J., Morrison, M. F., Reynolds, R. F., Glasser, D. B. & Strom, B. L. (2004). Comparative cardiac safety of low-dose thioridazine and low-dose haloperidol. *British Journal of Clinical Pharmacology*, *58*(1), 81-7.

Holbrook, S. Y. L., Garzan, A., Dennis, E. K., Shrestha, S. K. & Garneau-Tsodikova, S. (2017). Repurposing antipsychotic drugs into antifungal agents: Synergistic combinations of azoles and bromperidol derivatives in the treatment of various fungal infections. *European Journal of Medicinal Chemistry*, *139*, 12-21.

Howland, R. H. (2014). The comparative cardiac effects of haloperidol and quetiapine: parsing a review. *Journal of Psychosocial Nursing and Mental Health Services*, *52*(6), 23-6.

Huang, Y., Gao, F., Zhang, Y., Chen, Y., Wang, B., Zheng, Y. & Shi, G. (2012). N-n-Butyl haloperidol iodide inhibits the augmented Na+/Ca2+ exchanger currents and L-type Ca2+ current induced by hypoxia/reoxygenation or H2O2 in cardiomyocytes. *Biochemical and Biophysical Research Communications*, *421*(1), 86-90.

Huang, Z., Shi, G., Gao, F., Zhang, Y., Liu, X., Christopher, T. A., Lopez, B. & Ma, X. (2007). Effects of N-n-butyl haloperidol iodide on L-type calcium channels and intracellular free calcium in rat ventricular myocytes. *Biochemistry and Cell Biology*, *85*(2), 182-8.

Ifteni, P., Grudnikoff, E., Koppel, J., Kremen, N., Correll, C. U., Kane, J. M. & Manu, P. (2015). Haloperidol and sudden cardiac death in dementia: autopsy findings in psychiatric inpatients. *International Journal of Geriatric Psychiatry*, *30*(12), 1224-9.

Iwahashi, K. (1996). Significantly higher plasma haloperidol level during cotreatment with carbamazepine may herald cardiac change. *Clinical Neuropharmacology*, *19*(3), 267-70.

Jomphe, C., Lévesque, D. & Trudeau, L. E. (2003). Calcium-dependent, D2 receptor-independent induction of c-fos by haloperidol in dopamine neurons. *Naunyn-Schmiedeberg's Archives of Pharmacology, 367*(5), 480-9.

Khanzode, S. D., Mahakalkar, S. M., Belorkar, N. R., Kharkar, V. T. & Manekar, M. S. (1996). Effect of pre-treatment of some calcium channel blockers on catalepsy and stereotypic behaviour in rats. *Indian Journal of Physiology and Pharmacology, 40*(2), 159-62.

Kim, D. D., Lang, D. J., Warburton, D. E. R., Woodward, M. L., White, R. F., Barr, A. M., Honer, W. G. & Procyshyn, R. M. (2017). Heart-rate response to alpha2-adrenergic receptor antagonism by antipsychotics. *Clinical Autonomic Research: Official Journal of The Clinical Autonomic Research Society, 27*(6), 407-10.

Kim, H. S., Yumkham, S., Choi, J. H., Kim, E. K., Kim, Y. S., Ryu, S. H. & Suh, P. G. (2006). Haloperidol induces calcium ion influx via L-type calcium channels in hippocampal HN33 cells and renders the neurons more susceptible to oxidative stress. *Molecules and Cells, 22*(1), 51-7.

Kozlovskiĭ, V. L., Prakh'e, I. V. & Kenunen, O. G. (1996). The influence of calcium channel blockers on the effects of haloperidol and phenamine in mice and rats. *Experimental and Clinical Pharmacology, 59*(3), 12-5.

Lau, Y. S. & Gnegy, M. E. (1982). Chronic haloperidol treatment increased calcium-dependent phosphorylation in rat striatum. *Life Sciences, 30*(1), 21-8.

Lee, J., Rushlow, W. J. & Rajakumar, N. (2007). L-type calcium channel blockade on haloperidol-induced c-Fos expression in the striatum. *Neuroscience, 149*(3), 602-16.

Lencesova, L., Szadvari, I., Babula, P., Kubickova, J., Chovancova, B., Lopusna, K., Rezuchova, I., Novakova, Z., Krizanova, O. & Novakova, M. (2017). Disruption of dopamine D1/D2 receptor complex is involved in the function of haloperidol in cardiac H9c2 cells. *Life Sciences, 191*, 186-94.

Liu, Y., Xia, T., Wei, J., Liu, Q. & Li, X. (2017). Micropatterned co-culture of cardiac myocytes on fibrous scaffolds for predictive screening of drug cardiotoxicities. *Nanoscale, 9*(15), 4950-62.

Lu, B., Wang, B., Zhong, S., Zhang, Y., Gao, F., Chen, Y., Zheng, F. & Shi, G. (2016). N-n-butyl haloperidol iodide ameliorates hypoxia/ reoxygenation injury through modulating the LKB1/AMPK/ROS pathway in cardiac microvascular endothelial cells. *Oncotarget, 7*(23), 34800-10.

Machado, D., Pires, D., Perdigão, J., Couto, I., Portugal, I., Martins, M., Amaral, L., Anes, E. & Viveiros, M. (2016). Ion channel blockers as antimicrobial agents, efflux inhibitors, and enhancers of macrophage killing activity against drug resistant mycobacterium tuberculosis. *Public Library of Science One PLoS 1, 11*(2), e0149326.

Macht, M., Mull, A. C., McVaney, K. E., Caruso, E. H., Johnston, J. B., Gaither, J. B., Shupp, A. M., Marquez, K. D., Haukoos, J. S. & Colwell, C. B. (2014). Comparison of droperidol and haloperidol for use by paramedics: assessment of safety and effectiveness. *Prehospital Emergency Care: Official Journal of the National Association of EMS Physicians and the National Association of State EMS Directors, 18*(3), 375-80.

Medlin, R. P. Jr., Ransom, M. M., Watts, J. A. & Kline, J. A. (1996). Effect of ethanol, haloperidol, and lorazepam on cardiac conduction and contraction. *Journal of Cardiovascular Pharmacology, 28*(6), 792-8.

Metzger, E. & Friedman, R. (1993). Prolongation of the corrected QT and torsades de pointes cardiac arrhythmia associated with intravenous haloperidol in the medically ill. *Journal of Clinical Psychopharmacology, 13*(2), 128-32.

Metzger, E. & Friedman, R. (1993). Prolongation of the corrected QT and torsades de pointes cardiac arrhythmia associated with intravenous haloperidol in the medically ill. *Journal of Clinical Psycho-pharmacology, 13*(2), 128-32.

Meyer-Massetti, C., Cheng, C. M., Sharpe, B. A., Meier, C. R. & Guglielmo, B. J. (2010). The FDA extended warning for intravenous haloperidol and torsades de pointes: how should institutions respond? *Journal of Hospital Medicine, 5*(4), E8-16.

Meyer-Massetti, C., Vaerini, S., Rätz Bravo, A. E., Meier, C. R. & Guglielmo, B. J. (2011). Comparative safety of antipsychotics in the WHO pharmacovigilance database: the haloperidol case. *International Journal of Clinical Pharmacy*, *33*(5), 806-14.

Mörtl, D., Agneter, E., Krivanek, P., Koppatz, K. & Todt, H. (2003). Dual rate-dependent cardiac electrophysiologic effects of haloperidol: slowing of intraventricular conduction and lengthening of repolarization. *Journal of Cardiovascular Pharmacology*, *41*(6), 870-9.

Mörtl, D., Agneter, E., Krivanek, P., Koppatz, K. & Todt, H. (2003). Dual rate-dependent cardiac electrophysiologic effects of haloperidol: slowing of intraventricular conduction and lengthening of repolarization. *Journal of Cardiovascular Pharmacology*, *41*(6), 870-9.

Muzyk, A. J., Rayfield, A., Revollo, J. Y., Heinz, H. & Gagliardi, J. P. (2012). Examination of baseline risk factors for QTc interval prolongation in patients prescribed intravenous haloperidol. *Drug Safety*, *35*(7), 547-53.

Nade, V. S., Kawale, L. A. & Yadav, A. V. (2010). Protective effect of *Morus alba* leaves on haloperidol-induced orofacial dyskinesia and oxidative stress. *Pharmaceutical Biology*, *48*(1), 17-22.

Nalepa, I., Kreiner, G., Kowalska, M., Sanak, M. & Vetulani, J. (1999). Adrenergic receptors' responsiveness after acute and chronic treatment with haloperidol in the presence of calcium channel blockade. *Polish Journal of Pharmacology*, *51*(5), 377-83.

Neumaier, J. F. & Chavkin, C. (1989). Calcium-dependent displacement of haloperidol-sensitive sigma receptor binding in rat hippocampal slices following tissue depolarization. *Brain Research*, *500*(1-2), 215-22.

Novakova, M., Sedlakova, B., Sirova, M., Fialova, K. & Krizanova, O. (2010). Haloperidol increases expression of the inositol 1,4,5-trisphosphate receptors in rat cardiac atria, but not in ventricles. *General Physiology and Biophysics*, *29*(4), 381-9.

Palotás, A., Penke, B., Palotás, M., Kenderessy, A. S., Kemény, L., Kis, E., Vincze, G., Janka, Z. & Kálmán, J. (2004). Haloperidol attenuates beta-amyloid-induced calcium imbalance in human fibroblasts. *Skin Pharmacology and Physiology, 17*(4), 195-9.

Park, S. J., Jeong, J., Park, Y. U., Park, K. S., Lee, H., Lee, N., Kim, S. M., Kuroda, K., Nguyen, M. D., Kaibuchi, K. & Park, S. K. (2015). Disrupted-in-schizophrenia-1 (DISC1) Regulates Endoplasmic Reticulum Calcium Dynamics. *Scientific Reports, 5,* 8694.

Perera, J., Tan, J. H., Jeevathayaparan, S., Chakravarthi, S. & Haleagrahara, N. (2011). Neuroprotective effects of alpha lipoic Acid on haloperidol-induced oxidative stress in the rat brain. *Cell and Bioscience, 1*(1), 12.

Post, A., Holsboer, F. & Behl, C. (1998). Induction of NF-kappaB activity during haloperidol-induced oxidative toxicity in clonal hippocampal cells: suppression of NF-kappaB and neuroprotection by antioxidants. *The Journal of Neuroscience: The Official Journal of the Society for Neuroscience, 18*(20), 8236-46.

Raghu, K. G., Singh, R., Prathapan, A. & Yadav, G. K. (2009). Modulation of haloperidol induced electrophysiological alterations on cardiac action potential by various risk factors and gender difference. *Chemico-Biological Interactions, 180*(3), 454-9.

Raudenska, M., Gumulec, J., Babula, P., Stracina, T., Sztalmachova, M., Polanska, H., Adam, V., Kizek, R., Novakova, M. & Masarik, M. (2013). Haloperidol cytotoxicity and its relation to oxidative stress. *Mini Reviews in Medicinal Chemistry, 13*(14), 1993-8.

Reiriz, J., Ambrosio, S., Cobos, A., Ballarín, M., Tolosa, E. & Mahy, N. (1994). Dopaminergic function in rat brain after oral administration of calcium-channel blockers or haloperidol. A microdialysis study. *Journal of Neural Transmission. General Section, 95*(3), 195-207.

Rogoza, R. M., Fairfax, D. F., Henry, P., N-Marandi, S., Khan, R. F., Gupta, S. K. & Mishra, R. K. (2004). Electron spin resonance spectroscopy reveals alpha-phenyl-N-tert-butylnitrone spin-traps free radicals in rat striatum and prevents haloperidol-induced vacuous chewing movements in the rat model of human tardive dyskinesia. *Synapse, 54*(3), 156-63.

Sagara, Y. (1998). Induction of reactive oxygen species in neurons by haloperidol. *Journal of Neurochemistry*, *71*(3), 1002-12.

Satoh, Y., Sugiyama, A., Tamura, K. & Hashimoto, K. (2000). Effect of magnesium sulfate on the haloperidol-induced QT prolongation assessed in the canine *in vivo* model under the monitoring of monophasic action potential. *Japanese Circulation Journal*, *64*(6), 445-51.

Scharfetter, J. & Fischer, P. (2014). QTc prolongation induced by intravenous sedation with Haloperidol, Prothipendyl and Lorazepam. *Neuropsychiatrie: Klinik, Diagnostik, Therapie und Rehabilitation: Organ der Gesellschaft Österreichischer Nervenärzte und Psychiater*, *28*(1), 1-5.

Sczekan, S. R. & Strumwasser, F. (1996). Antipsychotic drugs block IP3-dependent Ca(2+)-release from rat brain microsomes. *Biological Psychiatry*, *40*(6), 497-502.

Seki, Y., Kato, T. A., Monji, A., Mizoguchi, Y., Horikawa, H., Sato-Kasai, M., Yoshiga, D. & Kanba, S. (2013). Pretreatment of aripiprazole and minocycline, but not haloperidol, suppresses oligodendrocyte damage from interferon-γ-stimulated microglia in co-culture model. *Schizophrenia Research*, *151*(1-3), 20-8.

Shi, G. G., Fang, H. & Zheng, J. H. (2001). Quaternary ammonium salt derivative of haloperidol inhibits KCl-induced calcium increase in rat aortic smooth muscle cells. *Acta Pharmacologica Sinica*, *22*(9), 837-40.

Shinoda, Y., Tagashira, H., Bhuiyan, M. S., Hasegawa, H., Kanai, H. & Fukunaga, K. (2016). Haloperidol aggravates transverse aortic constriction-induced heart failure via mitochondrial dysfunction. *Journal of Pharmacological Sciences*, *131*(3), 172-83.

Shivakumar, B. R. & Ravindranath, V. (1992). Oxidative stress induced by administration of the neuroleptic drug haloperidol is attenuated by higher doses of haloperidol. *Brain Research*, *595*(2), 256-62.

Stracina, T., Slaninova, I., Polanska, H., Axmanova, M., Olejnickova, V., Konecny, P., Masarik, M., Krizanova, O. & Novakova, M. (2015). Long-term haloperidol treatment prolongs QT interval and increases expression of sigma 1 and IP3 receptors in guinea pig hearts. *The Tohoku Journal of Experimental Medicine, 236*(3), 199-207.

Stylianou, M., Kulesskiy, E., Lopes, J. P., Granlund, M., Wennerberg, K. & Urban, C. F. (2014). Antifungal application of nonantifungal drugs. *Antimicrobial Agents and Chemotherapy, 58*(2), 1055-62.

Sugiyama, A., Satoh, Y. & Hashimoto, K. (2001). *In vivo* canine model comparison of cardiohemodynamic and electrophysiological effects of a new antipsychotic drug aripiprazole (OPC-14597) to haloperidol. *Toxicology and Applied Pharmacology, 173*(2), 120-8.

Tarabová, B., Nováková, M. & Lacinová, L. (2009). Haloperidol moderately inhibits cardiovascular L-type calcium current. *General Physiology and Biophysics, 28*(3), 249-59.

Tesar, G. E., Murray, G. B. & Cassem, N. H. (1985). Use of high-dose intravenous haloperidol in the treatment of agitated cardiac patients. *Journal of Clinical Psychopharmacology, 5*(6), 344-7.

Thaakur, S. R. & Jyothi, B. (2007). Effect of spirulina maxima on the haloperidol induced tardive dyskinesia and oxidative stress in rats. *Journal of Neural Transmission, 114*(9), 1217-25.

Thaakur, S. & Himabindhu, G. (2009). Effect of alpha lipoic acid on the tardive dyskinesia and oxidative stress induced by haloperidol in rats. *Journal of Neural Transmission, 116*(7), 807-14.

Vandael, E., Vandenberk, B., Vandenberghe, J., Spriet, I., Willems, R. & Foulon, V. (2016). Risk management of QTc-prolongation in patients receiving haloperidol: an epidemiological study in a University hospital in Belgium. *International Journal of Clinical Pharmacy, 38*(2), 310-20.

Wang, Z. & Wang, J. (2015). Sudden cardiac death after modified electroconvulsive therapy. *Shanghai Archives of Psychiatry, 27*(5), 315-8.

Warnier, M. J., Rutten, F. H., Souverein, P. C., de Boer, A., Hoes, A. W. & De Bruin, M. L. (2015). Are ECG monitoring recommendations before prescription of QT-prolonging drugs applied in daily practice? The example of haloperidol. *Pharmacoepidemiology and Drug Safety, 24*(7), 701-8.

Xiao, J. F. 1., Wang, C. Y., Huang, Y. P., Shen, J. X., Gao, F. F., Huang, Z. Q., Zheng, Y. S. & Shi, G. G. (2011). N-n-butyl haloperidol iodide preserves cardiomyocyte calcium homeostasis during hypoxia/ ischemia. *Cellular Physiology and Biochemistry: International Journal of Experimental Cellular Physiology, Biochemistry, and Pharmacology, 27*(5), 433-42.

Yang, C., Chen, Y., Tang, L. & Wang, Z. J. (2011). Haloperidol disrupts opioid-antinociceptive tolerance and physical dependence. *The Journal of Pharmacology and Experimental Therapeutics, 338*(1), 164-72.

Zhang, X. Y., Zhou, D. F., Shen, Y. C., Zhang, P. Y., Zhang, W. F., Liang, J., Chen, D. C., Xiu, M. H., Kosten, T. A. & Kosten, T. R. (2012). Effects of risperidone and haloperidol on superoxide dismutase and nitric oxide in schizophrenia. *Neuropharmacology, 62*(5-6), 1928-34.

Zhang, Y. M., Wang, C. Y., Zheng, F. C., Gao, F. F., Chen, Y. C., Huang, Z. Q., Xia, Z. Y., Irwin, M. G., Li, W. Q., Liu, X. P., Zheng, Y. S., Xu, H. & Shi, G. G. (2012). Effects of N-n-butyl haloperidol iodide on the rat myocardial sarcoplasmic reticulum Ca(2+)-ATPase during ischemia/reperfusion. *Biochemical and Biophysical Research Communications, 425*(2), 426-30.

Zhang, Y., Chen, G., Zhong, S., Zheng, F., Gao, F., Chen, Y., Huang, Z., Cai, W., Li, W., Liu, X., Zheng, Y., Xu, H. & Shi, G. (2013). N-n-butyl haloperidol iodide ameliorates cardiomyocytes hypoxia/ reoxygenation injury by extracellular calcium-dependent and - independent mechanisms. *Oxidative Medicine and Cellular Longevity, 2013*, 912310.

Zhou, Y., Zhang, Y., Gao, F., Guo, F., Wang, J., Cai, W., Chen, Y., Zheng, J. & Shi, G. (2010). N-n-butyl haloperidol iodide protects cardiac microvascular endothelial cells from hypoxia/reoxygenation injury by down-regulating Egr-1 expression. *Cellular Physiology and Biochemistry: International Journal of Experimental Cellular Physiology, Biochemistry, and Pharmacology, 26*(6), 839-48.

In: The Pharmacological Guide to Haloperidol   ISBN: 978-1-53614-700-1
Editor: Amor Harland   © 2019 Nova Science Publishers, Inc.

Chapter 4

A PHARMACOLOGICAL FMRI STUDY OF FACIAL EXPRESSIONS DURING HALOPERIDOL TREATMENT

Dorota Bartusik-Aebisher, David Aebisher and Adrian Truszkiewicz*
Faculty of Medicine, University of Rzeszów,
Rzeszów, Poland

ABSTRACT

The aim of this chapter is to present studies using functional magnetic resonance imaging (fMRI) to study aspects of the drug haloperidol on facial expressions. Emotion processing is often notable in neurodegenerative diseases such as schizophrenia and evaluated in cerebral blood flow response in diseased patients during facial emotion. This chapter describes facial expressions, salient in emotional behavior, that are used in conjunction with (fMRI) to investigate emotion processing during schizophrenia treated by haloperidol. The applications of blood-oxygen-level-dependent (BOLD) techniques to study

---

* Corresponding Author Email: dbartusik-aebisher@ur.edu.pl.

haloperidol responses and facial displays of emotions during haloperidol treatment are reviewed.

Keywords: fluorinated drug, haloperidol, functional magnetic resonance imaging

INTRODUCTION

Functional magnetic resonance (fMRI), is a relatively new study of brain activity. Today, the fMRI test allows, among others carefully assess the type of cancer, quickly diagnose multiple sclerosis and Alzheimer's disease, and also explain the mystery of the human mind, including phantom pain in patients with amputated limbs. The fMRI test, or functional magnetic resonance imaging, is a non-invasive method of imaging the activity of the human brain during normal functioning, using the phenomenon of changing the level of blood oxygenation.

Structural resonance is based on the magnetic properties of the atoms that make up the body's cells. When atoms are placed in an external magnetic field, they are subjected to an electromagnetic pulse of radio frequency. As a consequence, physical processes are initiated, thanks to which the atomic nuclei become magnetized and become the source of the electromagnetic field themselves. The energy emitted by them is received by the computer, given to the analysis and processed into the image. It should be mentioned that the atoms of cells have different magnetic properties, therefore each of them returns a signal of a different intensity. Thanks to this, it is possible to distinguish different tissues from one another those that are healthy and pathologically altered. Pain is an unpleasant sensory and emotional experience that accompanies the existing or threatening tissue damage or is only related to such damage. A characteristic feature of pain includes two components: sensory, associated with the perception of pain, which allows its location, and emotional, associated with the psychological response of a patient with a painful stimulus. This second component of pain is highly subjective; hence the experience of pain is different in individual patients. It is thought that pain always occurs when it is reported by the patient.

Most painkillers can be included in one of the following groups: non-opioid analgesics: paracetamol and non-steroidal anti-inflammatory drugs; weak opioids; strong opioids; supplementary medicines. It is recommended to associate drugs with different mechanisms of action (administration of non-opioid analgesics with opioids). It is not recommended to simultaneously administer several drugs with the same mechanism of action. The combination of strong opioids has not yet been unequivocally evaluated, although in some experimental and clinical studies an improvement in analgesia has been demonstrated, without the severity of side effects, when morphine is combined with percutaneous fentanyl, morphine with methadone and oxycodone with morphine. Combination of sustained and immediate release preparations (sustained-release morphine and short-acting morphine, percutaneous fentanyl or percutaneous buprenorphine with rapid-release morphine in the treatment of breakthrough pain) is recommended.

During the last years, an interest and knowledge of fMRI has occurred in research and in the clinic. Significant advances have been made in the general understanding of fMRI to monitor diagnosis and treatment of neurodegenerative diseases. The purpose of this chapter is to present update information about the potential of fMRI and facial pain.

Studies by Fakara and coworkers present report on emotional processing that occurs in schizophrenic patients (Fakra et al. 2008). They present a specific pattern of emotional responding that usually includes deficits in emotional expressiveness, increased feelings of unpleasant emotion but decreased feelings of pleasant emotion, and increased physiological reactivity (Fakra et al. 2008). The paper present completed research on emotional states of fear, sadness, anger, joy, and disgust were induced, as well as a neutral baseline state and facial expression (Fakra et al. 2008). The schizophrenics and depressives patients are often characterized by different quantitative, qualitative, and dysfunctions (Wölwer et al. 1996; Gaebel and Wölwer 1992), thus fMRI can be employ to monitor neurodegenerative disorders.

Haloperidol is an example of a fluorinated drug used for to treat schizophrenia to salient various features for neutral and happy (Fakra et al. 2009; Williams et al. 2003). The aim of study performed by Kucharska-Pietura and coworkers was to assess social cognition in schizophrenia inpatients being treated with first-generation antipsychotic drugs such as haloperidol (Kucharska-Pietura et al. 2012). Patients with schizophrenia show impairments in social information processing, such as recognizing facial emotions and face identity (Barkhof et al. 2015). The aim of this study was to explore whether these impairments represent specific deficits or are part of a more general cognitive dysfunction (Barkhof et al. 2015). There is no deficit in identifying facial emotions in schizophrenia. There may, however, be a deficit in judging emotional intensity. The impairment found in naming familiar faces is consistent with other evidence of semantic memory impairment in the disorder (Pomarol-Clotet et al. 2010). Impairment in the specificity of emotion identification may lead to misunderstanding of social communication and may underlie difficulties in social adjustment experienced by people with schizophrenia (Schneider et al. 2006). The behavioral deficit in face emotion processing is mirrored in an underlying neural impairment (McCleery et al. 2015).

Many studies underline the role of dysfunctional neural networks as the basis of disturbed social interactions in early schizophrenia (Reske et al. 2009). Patients showed reduced blood oxygenation level-dependent (BOLD) activation in the fusiform, inferior frontal, middle temporal and middle occipital gyrus as well as in the amygdala. These results suggest that problems in facial affect recognition in schizophrenia may represent flow-on effects of a generalized deficit in early visual processing (Johnston et al. 2005). Relative to control subjects, the patients demonstrated (1) significantly greater activation of the left hippocampus while viewing all three facial expressions and (2) increased right amygdala activation during the initial presentation of fearful and neutral facial expressions. In schizophrenia, hippocampal and amygdala activity is elevated during the passive viewing of human faces (Holt et al. 2006). In terms of brain activity, motor learning may be less efficient or slower in the patients than in healthy subjects (Kodama et al. 2001).

Stable dysfunctions which are unaffected by therapy and symptom improvement were found in cortico-limbic regions crucially involved in emotion processing. They presumably reflect patients' difficulties in emotion regulation and emotional memory processes. However, therapy-related activation changes were also observed and demonstrate efficacy of antipsychotic therapy on improving emotion functionality (Reske et al. 2007). This is the first time that brain activation changes in a seriously disabled group of patients with schizophrenia can be associated clearly with psychological rather than pharmacological therapy (Wykes et al. 2002). The study by Stip and coworkers investigates changes in cerebral activation related to emotion processing in schizophrenia patients. Using fMRI, brain activation in 12 schizophrenia patients during passive viewing of sad film excerpts was studied before and after a median of 5.5-month treatment with quetiapine. Random-effects 'paired sample t-test' analyses of brain activation before quetiapine (contrast=sad-neutral, before-after) revealed significant activation in the brainstem (Stip et al. 2005). During working memory performance, parietal hypoactivations were accompanied by poorer performance in patients. A hyperfrontality emerged in the ventrolateral prefrontal cortex. Hence, results point to a dysfunctional ventrolateral prefrontal-parietal network during working memory in patients, suggesting impairments in basic functions such as retrieval, storage and maintenance. The brain activation pattern of this large and significant sample of first-episode schizophrenia patients indicates an imbalanced system failing to adjust the amount of brain activity required in the cerebral network involved in attention and working memory (Schneider et al. 2007). These results point to a dysfunction in cerebral circuits relevant for emotion processing already prominent in adolescent schizophrenia patients. Regions affected by a decrease in activation are related to visual and face processing, similar to deficits reported in adult patients. These changes are accompanied by hyperactivations in areas related to emotion regulation and attribution, possibly reflecting compensatory mechanisms (Seiferth et al. 2009). Most studies focused on emotional face processes, whereas non-emotional face processing received less attention (Kronbichler et al. 2018). During the task period, subjects were asked to view happy (or angry/disgusting/sad) and neutral faces simultaneously presented every 3s and to judge which face was more emotional (positive or negative face discrimination). Imaging data were investigated in voxel-by-voxel basis for single-group analysis and for between-group analysis according to the random effect model using Statistical Parametric Mapping (Kosaka et al. 2002). BOLD response was significantly correlated with increased negative affect across multiple measures (Tso et al. 2015). Patients with schizophrenia showed abnormalities in the social brain neural circuit during facial emotion processing, in comparison with nonpsychotic siblings and healthy controls. The current findings support the universality of emotion perception impairments in schizophrenia, and also suggest that facial emotion perception might be a potential endophenotype of schizophrenia (Villalta-Gil et al. 2013; Li et al. 2012). Schizophrenia patients appear to be characterized by amygdalar hyperresponsiveness to negative and positive facial expressions on an automatic processing level. Heightened automatic amygdala responsivity could be involved in the development and maintenance of negative symptoms in schizophrenia (Rauch et al. 2010). Functional MRI was used to examine neural activity in 25 patients with diagnosis of schizophrenia while they participated in a face processing task, which involved viewing videos of angry and neutral facial expressions, and a non-biological baseline condition. Given that the anterior cingulate plays a role in processing negative emotion, weaker deactivation of this region in patients while viewing faces may contribute to an increased perception of social threat. Future studies examining the neurobiology of social cognition in schizophrenia using fMRI may help establish targets for treatment interventions (Mothersill et al. 2014). Functional magnetic resonance imaging tasks using the pictures of mild and intense facial emotions of fear or happiness (Surguladze et al. 2011). A marked underrecruitment of the amygdala, accompanied by a substantial limitation in activation throughout a ventral temporal-basal ganglion-prefrontal cortex "social brain" system may be central to the difficulties patients experience when processing facial emotion (Li et al. 2010). Results suggest that activation abnormalities during facial emotion perception are manifestations of the genetic liability to schizophrenia, and may be accompanied by compensatory mechanisms in relatives. Studying mechanisms in nonpsychotic relatives is a valuable way to examine effects of the unexpressed genetic liability to schizophrenia on the brain and behavior (Spilka et al. 2015). Patients showed a differential response to verbal and facial feedback in the rostral cingulate zone, whereas healthy controls did not differ between modalities. Furthermore, activation in the rostral cingulate zone following facial feedback was negatively related to severity of the disease as expressed by the scores on positive symptom subscale of the Positive and Negative Syndrome Scale. Both findings point in the direction of a specific deficit in patients which is related to the emotional impact of external feedback (van der Veen et al. 2013). In contrast, controls activated a much larger set of regions for happy faces, including areas thought to underlie recollection-based memory retrieval and in novelty detection. This study demonstrates that, despite an overall lower memory accuracy, emotional memory is intact in schizophrenia, although emotion-specific differences in brain activation exist, possibly reflecting different strategies (Sergerie et al. 2010). Schizophrenia patients show reduced insula responsiveness to micro-expressions but not macro-expressions of disgust compared to healthy controls. In patients, low agreeableness was associated with stronger insula response to micro- and macro-expressions of disgust. Patients with a strong tendency to feel uncomfortable with social interactions appear to be characterized by a high sensitivity for facial expression signaling social rejection. Given the associations of insula responsiveness to covert disgust expression with low agreeableness in healthy individuals, insula responsiveness to expressions of disgust might be in general a neural marker of the personality trait of agreeableness (Lindner et al. 2014). Results indicate the effectiveness of a dynamic functional localizer at identifying regions of interest associated with face perception and emotion recognition in schizophrenia (Arnold et al. 2016). Results confirm previous findings of left prefrontal hyperactivity contrasted with hypoactivity in right prefrontal cortex (Wolf et al. 2011). During facial affect processing, patients show overactivation in subcortical regions and under activation in prefrontal regions of the facial affect processing network, consistent with the notion of reduced emotional regulation. By contrast, overactivation within visual processing regions coupled with reduced engagement of facial affect processing regions points to abnormal visual integration was observed (Delvecchio et al. 2013). Results indicate an association between impaired extrastriate visual processing of facial fear and negative symptoms, which may underlie the previously reported difficulties of patients with negative symptoms in the recognition of facial fear (Michalopoulou et al. 2008). Results indicate that altered connectivity in a visual-limbic subnetwork during emotional face processing may be a functional connectomic intermediate phenotype for schizophrenia. The phenotype is reliable, task specific, related to trait anxiety, and associated with manifest illness. These data encourage the further investigation of this phenotype in clinical and pharmacologic studies (Cao et al. 2016). Neuroimaging studies of emotional response in schizophrenia have mainly used visual (faces) paradigms and shown globally reduced brain activity. None of these studies have used an auditory paradigm (Sanjuan et al. 2007). Studies suggest that the affective response is impaired in both schizophrenia and adolescent offspring of schizophrenia patients. Here using fMRI they assessed the intra-amygdala response to positive, negative, and neutral valenced faces in a group of controls (with no family history of psychosis) and offspring of schizophrenia parents. Subjects performed an affective continuous performance task during which they continually appraised whether the affect signaled by a face on a given trial was the same or different from the previous trial (regardless of facial identity) (Barbour et al. 2010). Blood oxygenation level-dependent changes were contrasted for task compared with a scrambled face baseline (blocked analysis) and for the appearance of each of the following 4 target expressions compared with neutral faces (event related): happy, sad, anger, and fear. The percentage of signal change for each contrast and performance and clinical symptom severity ratings. Patients showed reduced limbic activation compared with controls for the emotion identification task. Abnormal amygdala activation in schizophrenia in response to presentation of fearful faces is paradoxically associated with failure to recognize the emotion and with more severe flat affect. This finding suggests that flat affect in schizophrenia relates to overstimulation of the limbic system (Gur et al. 2007). The effects of D2 dopamine receptor agonist, bromocriptine (BROMO), and antagonist, haloperidol (HPD), on brain activity were investigated in rats by functional magnetic resonance imaging. T_2^*-weighted signal intensity was increased in the hypothalamus at 120 min after acute administration of BROMO, and in the ventral posterior and dorsomedial nuclei of the thalamus from 30 to 120 min. These results suggest that the D2 receptor agonist increased the activity of the thalamic nuclei and the hypothalamus (Hagino et al. 1998). fMRI is a well-established, non-invasive technique for mapping the working brain. Yet imaging of subcortical regions has proven to be difficult. We studied 40 subjects performing a unilateral self-paced finger-tapping task. This study emphasizes the possibility of investigating subcortical brain activation in patients with schizophrenia. The results of the present study outline the importance of further fMRI studies to investigate interindividual activation differences under different conditions especially focusing on basal ganglia (Müller et al. 2002). Healthy participants took an acute dose of amphetamine, haloperidol, or placebo. fMRI was used to measure the BOLD signal while they carried out an aversive conditioning task, using cutaneous electrical stimulation as the unconditioned stimulus and yellow and blue circles as conditioned stimulus (CS+ and CS-, respectively). The results provide the first demonstration that the modulation of dopamine transmission affects both the physiological correlates and PE related BOLD activity during aversive learning (Menon et al. 2007). In the presence of haloperidol, reduced correlation was observed between the substantia nigra and several brain regions, notably the cingulate and prefrontal cortices, posterodorsal hippocampus, ventral pallidum, and motor cortex. Haloperidol induced focal changes in functional connectivity were found to be the most strongly associated with ascending dopamine projections (Gass et al. 2013). Here, they used a pharmacological challenge in combination with functional magnetic resonance imaging to investigate the impact of dopaminergic receptor blockade on whole brain functional connectivity in twenty healthy human subjects. Our findings might also aid in interpreting alterations in more complex states, such as those seen psychiatric conditions and their treatment (Haaker et al. 2016). The regional neuronal changes taking place in the early and late stages of antipsychotic treatment are still not well characterized in humans. In addition, it is not known whether these regional changes are predictive of or are correlated with treatment response. Using PET with ^{15}O, we evaluated the time course of regional cerebral blood flow patterns generated by a first (haloperidol) and a second (olanzapine) generation antipsychotic drug in patients with schizophrenia during a 6-week treatment trial. As hypothesized, we observed regional cerebral blood flow changes that were common to both the drugs, implicating cortico-subcortical and limbic neuronal networks in antipsychotic action (Lahti et al. 2009).

CONCLUSION

The use of fMRI facial expressions of pain during neurodegenerative diseases is often monitored. The potential of fMRI in this matter is recognized by medicine research.

ACKNOWLEDGMENTS

Dorota Bartusik-Aebisher acknowledges support from the National Center of Science NCN (New drug delivery systems-MRI study, Grant OPUS-13 number 2017/25/B/ST4/02481).

REFERENCES

Arnold, A. E., Iaria, G., Goghari, V. M. (2016). Efficacy of identifying neural components in the face and emotion processing system in schizophrenia using a dynamic functional localizer. *Psychiatry research. Neuroimaging*, 248:55-63.

Barbour, T., Murphy, E., Pruitt, P., Eickhoff, S. B., Keshavan, M. S., Rajan, U., Zajac-Benitez, C., Diwadkar, V. A. (2010). Reduced intra-amygdala activity to positively valenced faces in adolescent schizophrenia offspring. *Schizophrenia Research*, 123(2-3):126-36.

Barkhof, E., de Sonneville, L. M. J., Meijer, C. J., de Haan, L. (2015). Specificity of facial emotion recognition impairments in patients with multi-episode schizophrenia. *Schizophrenia Research. Cognition*, 2(1):12-19.

Cao, H., Bertolino, A., Walter, H., Schneider, M., Schäfer, A., Taurisano, P., Blasi, G., Haddad, L., Grimm, O., Otto, K., Dixson, L., Erk, S., Mohnke, S., Heinz, A., Romanczuk-Seiferth, N., Mühleisen, T. W., Mattheisen, M., Witt, S. H., Cichon, S., Noethen, M., Rietschel, M., Tost, H., Meyer-Lindenberg, A. (2016). Altered functional subnetwork during emotional face processing: a potential intermediate phenotype for schizophrenia. *Journal of the American Medical Association Psychiatry*, 73(6):598-605.

Delvecchio, G., Sugranyes, G., Frangou, S. (2013). Evidence of diagnostic specificity in the neural correlates of facial affect processing in bipolar disorder and schizophrenia: a meta-analysis of functional imaging studies. *Psychological Medicine*, 43(3):553-69.

Fakra, E., Khalfa, S., Da Fonseca, D., Besnier, N., Delaveau, P., Azorin, J. M., Blin, O. (2008). Effect of risperidone versus haloperidol on emotional responding in schizophrenic patients. *Psychopharmacology*, 200(2):261-72.

Fakra, E., Salgado-Pineda, P., Besnier, N., Azorin, J. M., Blin, O. (2009). Risperidone versus haloperidol for facial affect recognition in schizophrenia: findings from a randomised study. *The World Journal of Biological Psychiatry: The Official Journal of the World Federation of Societies of Biological Psychiatry*, 10(4 Pt 3):719-28.

Gaebel, W. and Wölwer, W. (1992). Facial expression and emotional face recognition in schizophrenia and depression. *European Archives of Psychiatry and Clinical Neuroscience*, 242(1):46-52.

Gass, N., Schwarz, A. J., Sartorius, A., Cleppien, D., Zheng, L., Schenker, E., Risterucci, C., Meyer-Lindenberg, A., Weber-Fahr, W. (2013). Haloperidol modulates midbrain-prefrontal functional connectivity in the rat brain. *European Neuropsychopharmacology: The Journal of the European College of Neuropsychopharmacology*, 23(10):1310-9.

Gur, R. E., McGrath, C., Chan, R. M., Schroeder, L., Turner, T., Turetsky, B. I., Kohler, C., Alsop, D., Maldjian, J., Ragland, J. D., Gur, R. C. (2002). An fMRI study of facial emotion processing in patients with schizophrenia. *The American Journal of Psychiatry*, 159(12):1992-9.

Gur, R. E., Loughead, J., Kohler, C. G., Elliott, M. A., Lesko, K., Ruparel, K., Wolf, D. H., Bilker, W. B., Gur, R. C. (2007). Limbic activation associated with misidentification of fearful faces and flat affect in schizophrenia. *Archives of General Psychiatry*, 64(12):1356-66.

Haaker, J., Menz, M. M., Fadai, T., Eippert, F., Büchel, C. (2016). Dopaminergic receptor blockade changes a functional connectivity network centred on the amygdala. *Human Brain Mapping*, 37(11):4148-57.

Hagino, H., Tabuchi, E., Kurachi, M., Saitoh, O., Sun, Y., Kondoh, T., Ono, T., Torii, K. (1998). Effects of D2 dopamine receptor agonist and antagonist on brain activity in the rat assessed by functional magnetic resonance imaging. *Brain Research*, 813(2):367-73.

Holt, D. J., Kunkel, L., Weiss, A. P., Goff, D. C., Wright, C. I., Shin, L. M., Rauch, S. L., Hootnick, J., Heckers, S. (2006). Increased medial temporal lobe activation during the passive viewing of emotional and neutral facial expressions in schizophrenia. *Schizophrenia Research*, 82(2-3):153-62.

Johnston, P. J., Stojanov, W., Devir, H., Schall, U. (2005). Functional MRI of facial emotion recognition deficits in schizophrenia and their electrophysiological correlates. *The European Journal of Neuroscience*, 22(5):1221-32.

Kodama, S., Fukuzako, H., Fukuzako, T., Kiura, T., Nozoe, S., Hashiguchi, T., Yamada, K., Takenouchi, K., Takigawa, M., Nakabeppu, Y., Nakajo, M. (2001). Aberrant brain activation following motor skill learning in schizophrenic patients as shown by functional magnetic resonance imaging. *Psychological Medicine,* 31(6):1079-88.

Kosaka, H., Omori, M., Murata, T., Iidaka, T., Yamada, H., Okada, T., Takahashi, T., Sadato, N., Itoh, H., Yonekura, Y., Wada, Y. (2002). Differential amygdala response during facial recognition in patients with schizophrenia: an fMRI study. *Schizophrenia Research,* 57(1):87-95.

Kronbichler, L., Stelzig-Schöler, R., Pearce, B. G., Tschernegg, M., Said-Yürekli, S., Reich, L. A., Weber, S., Aichhorn, W., Kronbichler, M. (2018). Schizophrenia and Category-Selectivity in the Brain: Normal for Faces but Abnormal for Houses. *Frontiers in Psychiatry,* 9:47.

Kucharska-Pietura, K., Mortimer, A., Tylec, A., Czernikiewicz, A. (2012). Social cognition and visual perception in schizophrenia inpatients treated with first-and second-generation antipsychotic drugs. *Clinical Schizophrenia and Related Psychoses,* 6(1):14-20.

Lahti, A. C., Weiler, M. A., Holcomb, H. H., Tamminga, C. A., Cropsey, K. L. (2009). Modulation of limbic circuitry predicts treatment response to antipsychotic medication: a functional imaging study in schizophrenia. *Neuropsychopharmacology: Official Publication of the American College of Neuropsychopharmacology,* 34(13):2675-90.

Lindner, C., Dannlowski, U., Walhöfer, K., Rödiger, M., Maisch, B., Bauer, J., Ohrmann, P., Lencer, R., Zwitserlood, P., Kersting, A., Heindel, W., Arolt, V., Kugel, H., Suslow, T. (2014). Social alienation in schizophrenia patients: association with insula responsiveness to facial expressions of disgust. *Public Library of Science One PLoS 1,* 9(1):e85014.

Li, H. J., Chan, R. C., Gong, Q. Y., Liu, Y., Liu, S. M., Shum, D., Ma, Z. L. (2012). Facial emotion processing in patients with schizophrenia and their non-psychotic siblings: a functional magnetic resonance imaging study. *Schizophrenia Research,* 134(2-3):143-50.

Li, H., Chan, R. C., McAlonan, G. M., Gong, Q. Y. (2010). Facial emotion processing in schizophrenia: a meta-analysis of functional neuroimaging data. *Schizophrenia Bulletin,* 36(5):1029-39.

McCleery, A., Lee, J., Joshi, A., Wynn, J. K., Hellemann, G. S., Green, M. F. (2015). Meta-analysis of face processing event-related potentials in schizophrenia. *Biological Psychiatry*, 77(2):116-26.

Menon, M., Jensen, J., Vitcu, I., Graff-Guerrero, A., Crawley, A., Smith, M. A., Kapur, S. (2007). Temporal difference modeling of the blood-oxygen level dependent response during aversive conditioning in humans: effects of dopaminergic modulation. *Biological Psychiatry*, 62(7):765-72.

Michalopoulou, P. G., Surguladze, S., Morley, L. A., Giampietro, V. P., Murray, R. M., Shergill, S. S. (2008). Facial fear processing and psychotic symptoms in schizophrenia: functional magnetic resonance imaging study. *The British Journal of Psychiatry: The Journal of Mental Science*, 192(3):191-6.

Mothersill, O., Morris, D. W., Kelly, S., Rose, E. J., Bokde, A., Reilly, R., Gill, M., Corvin, A. P., Donohoe, G. (2014). Altered medial prefrontal activity during dynamic face processing in schizophrenia spectrum patients. *Schizophrenia Research*, 157(1-3):225-30.

Müller, J. L., Röder, C., Schuierer, G., Klein, H. E. (2002). Subcortical overactivation in untreated schizophrenic patients: a functional magnetic resonance image finger-tapping study. *Psychiatry and Clinical Neurosciences*, 56(1):77-84.

Pomarol-Clotet, E., Hynes, F., Ashwin, C., Bullmore, E. T., McKenna, P. J., Laws, K. R. (2010). Facial emotion processing in schizophrenia: a non-specific neuropsychological deficit? *Psychological Medicine*, 40(6):911-9.

Rauch, A. V., Reker, M., Ohrmann, P., Pedersen, A., Bauer, J., Dannlowski, U., Harding, L., Koelkebeck, K., Konrad, C., Kugel, H., Arolt, V., Heindel, W., Suslow, T. (2010). Increased amygdala activation during automatic processing of facial emotion in schizophrenia. *Psychiatry Research*, 182(3):200-6.

Reske, M., Kellermann, T., Habel, U., Jon Shah, N., Backes, V., von Wilmsdorff, M., Stöcker, T., Gaebel, W., Schneider, F. (2007). Stability of emotional dysfunctions? A long-term fMRI study in first-episode schizophrenia. *Journal of Psychiatric Research*, 41(11):918-27.

Reske, M., Habel, U., Kellermann, T., Backes, V., Jon Shah, N., von Wilmsdorff, M., Gaebel, W., Zilles, K., Schneider, F. (2009). Differential brain activation during facial emotion discrimination in first-episode schizophrenia. *Journal of Psychiatric Research*, 43(6):592-9.

Sanjuan, J., Lull, J. J., Aguilar, E. J., Martí-Bonmatí, L., Moratal, D., Gonzalez, J. C., Robles, M., Keshavan, M. S. (2007). Emotional words induce enhanced brain activity in schizophrenic patients with auditory hallucinations. *Psychiatry Research*, 154(1):21-9.

Schneider, F., Habel, U., Reske, M., Kellermann, T., Stöcker, T., Shah, N. J., Zilles, K., Braus, D. F., Schmitt, A., Schlösser, R., Wagner, M., Frommann, I., Kircher, T., Rapp, A., Meisenzahl, E., Ufer, S., Ruhrmann, S., Thienel, R., Sauer, H., Henn, F. A., Gaebel, W. (2007). Neural correlates of working memory dysfunction in first-episode schizophrenia patients: an fMRI multi-center study. *Schizophrenia Research*, 89(1-3):198-210.

Schneider, F., Gur, R. C., Koch, K., Backes, V., Amunts, K., Shah, N. J., Bilker, W., Gur, R. E., Habel, U. (2006). Impairment in the specificity of emotion processing in schizophrenia. *The American Journal of Psychiatry*, 163(3):442-7.

Seiferth, N. Y., Pauly, K., Kellermann, T., Shah, N. J., Ott, G., Herpertz-Dahlmann, B., Kircher, T., Schneider, F., Habel, U. (2009). Neuronal correlates of facial emotion discrimination in early onset schizophrenia. *Neuropsychopharmacology: Official Publication of The American College of Neuropsychopharmacology*, 34(2):477-87.

Sergerie, K., Armony, J. L., Menear, M., Sutton, H., Lepage, M. (2010). Influence of emotional expression on memory recognition bias in schizophrenia as revealed by fMRI. *Schizophrenia Bulletin*, 36(4):800-10.

Spilka, M. J., Arnold, A. E., Goghari, V. M. (2015). Functional activation abnormalities during facial emotion perception in schizophrenia patients and nonpsychotic relatives. *Schizophrenia Research*, 168(1-2):330-7.

Stip, E., Fahim, C., Mancini-Marïe, A., Bentaleb, L. A., Mensour, B., Mendrek, A., Beauregard, M. (2005). Restoration of frontal activation during a treatment with quetiapine: an fMRI study of blunted affect in schizophrenia. *Progress in Neuro-psychopharmacology and Biological Psychiatry*, 29(1):21-6.

Surguladze, S. A., Chu, E. M., Marshall, N., Evans, A., Anilkumar, A. P., Timehin, C., McDonald, C., Ecker, C., Phillips, M. L., David, A. S. (2011). Emotion processing in schizophrenia: fMRI study of patients treated with risperidone long-acting injections or conventional depot medication. *Journal of Psychopharmacology / British Association for Psychopharmacology*, 25(6):722-33.

Tso, I. F., Fang, Y., Phan, K. L., Welsh, R. C., Taylor, S. F. (2015). Abnormal GABAergic function and face processing in schizophrenia: A pharmacologic-fMRI study. *Schizophrenia Research*, 168(1-2):338-44.

Van der Veen, F. M., Röder, C. H., Smits, M. (2013). Feedback processing in schizophrenia: effects of affective value and remedial action. *Psychiatry Research*, 213(2):108-14.

Villalta-Gil, V., Meléndez-Pérez, I., Russell, T., Surguladze, S., Radua, J., Fusté, M., Stephan-Otto, C., Haro, J. M. (2013). Functional similarity of facial emotion processing between people with a first episode of psychosis and healthy subjects. *Schizophrenia Research*, 149(1-3):35-41.

Williams, L. M., Loughland, C. M., Green, M. J., Harris, A. W., Gordon, E. (2003). Emotion perception in schizophrenia: an eye movement study comparing the effectiveness of risperidone vs. haloperidol. *Psychiatry Research*, 120(1):13-27.

Wolf, C., Linden, S., Jackson, M. C., Healy, D., Baird, A., Linden, D. E., Thome, J. (2011). Brain activity supporting working memory accuracy in patients with paranoid schizophrenia: a functional magnetic resonance imaging study. *Neuropsychobiology*, 64(2):93-101.

Wölwer, W., Streit, M., Polzer, U., Gaebel, W. (1996). Facial affect recognition in the course of schizophrenia. *European Archives of Psychiatry and Clinical Neuroscience*, 246(3):165-70.

Wykes, T., Brammer, M., Mellers, J., Bray, P., Reeder, C., Williams, C., Corner, J. (2002). Effects on the brain of a psychological treatment: cognitive remediation therapy: functional magnetic resonance imaging in schizophrenia. *The British Journal of Psychiatry: The Journal of Mental Science*, 181:144-52.

In: The Pharmacological Guide to Haloperidol   ISBN: 978-1-53614-700-1
Editor: Amor Harland   © 2019 Nova Science Publishers, Inc.

Chapter 5

THE USE OF fMRI
TO IDENTIFY BIOMARKERS DURING
HALOPERIDOL TREATMENT

David Aebisher, Dorota Bartusik-Aebisher*
and Adrian Truszkiewicz
Faculty of Medicine, University of Rzeszów, Rzeszów, Poland

ABSTRACT

Functional magnetic resonance imaging (fMRI) has been used to
probe brain biomarkers of healthy individuals and patients during
haloperidol treatments. A current review is presented to examine the
sensitivity of fMRI in behavioral testing performed for detecting early
neurodegenerative changes related to all diseases treated by haloperidol.
This chapter will also cover a literature analysis of the use of haloperidol,
in which studies indicate a limit may exist for haloperidol efficacy; values
above this limit seem not to provide any supplementary clinical
improvement and may even reduce therapeutic effect.

---

* Corresponding Author Email: daebisher@ur.edu.pl.

Keywords: haloperidol, biomarker, functional magnetic resonance imaging

INTRODUCTION

A biomarker is an indication which may indicate the presence of a disease state, or physiological or mental disorder. Biomarkers also controls the body's response to healing. In the past decade, magnetic resonance imaging (MRI) has reveolutionized the practice of medicine. MRI provides more contrast for most imaging problems in the brain. This is due both to the multiplicity of variables on which the MR signal depends (e.g., proton density, T_1 and T_2 and to the wealth of pulsing sequences available (e.g., T_1 or T_2 -weighted spin echo, inversion recovery and gradient echo sequences. In addition, MRI can easily produce images in plane. MRI is safer than CT. Even the contrast agent used for MRI (Gadolinium DTPA) is safer than the iodinated contrast agent used in CT. MRI has become the preffered radiologist technique for imaging the brain. MRI is a computered based imaging modality. The generation of an MR image requires the combination of spatial and intensity information. Studies of cerebral tumors have provided a useful clinical test for the development of faster sequences. MRI of central nervous system tumours has eveloped rapidly since the first publication on the subject on 1980 (Hawkes et al. 1980). Functional MRI was used to determine the acute blood oxygen level dependent effect (BOLD) of neuroleptic drugs (Brassen et al. 2016). The results are used for studying cerebral psychopharmacological effects (Brassen et al. 2016). Research of the effects of haloperidol was developed to study the motor function in 20 healthy men. They observed an effect of Haloperidol compared with placebo, with increased task-related recruitment of posterior cingulate and precentral gyri (Goozee et al. 2017). Brain function in schizophrenia was investigated by means of a simple motor task with a self-generated left-hand sequential finger opposition using a whole-brain high-speed functional imaging technique (Braus et al. 1999). Healthy participants received an acute oral dose of haloperidol, aripiprazole or placebo, and then performed an active aversive conditioning task with aversive and neutral events presented as sounds, while BOLD fMRI was carried out (Bolstad et al. 2015). The regional neuronal changes taking place in the early and late stages of antipsychotic treatment are still not well characterized in humans (Lahti et al. 2009). Antipsychotic drugs target neurotransmitter systems that play key roles in working memory. Elucidating the mechanisms by which antipsychotic medications alter brain activation underlying cognition is essential to advance pharmacological treatment of various disorders (Goozee et al. 2016; Cole et al. 2013). The effects of haloperidol on brain activity were investigated in rats by functional magnetic resonance imaging. T2* weighted signal intensity was increased in the hypothalamus. These results suggest that the D2 receptor agonist increased the activity of the thalamic nuclei and the hypothalamus (Hagino et al. 1998). fMRI is a non-invasive technique for mapping the working brain. Using a fingertapping task, imaging of subcortical regions has proven to be difficult (Müller and Klein 2000). fMRI is a well established, non-invasive technique for mapping the working brain. This study emphasizes the possibility of investigating subcortical brain activation in patients with schizophrenia. The results of the present study outline the importance of further fMRI studies to investigate interindividual activation differences under different conditions especially focusing on basal ganglia (Müller et al. 2002). MRI studies suggest that antipsychotic -treated patients with schizophrenia show a decrease in gray-matter volumes (Vernon et al. 2012). Healthy participants received an acute oral dose of haloperidol, aripiprazole or placebo before performing an executive functioning task while BOLD fMRI was carried out. The image analysis yielded a strong task-related BOLD-fMRI response within each group. An uncorrected between-group analysis showed that aripiprazole challenge resulted in stronger activation in the frontal and temporal gyri and the putamen compared with haloperidol challenge, but after correcting for multiple testing there was no significant group difference (Bolstad et al. 2015; Madularu et al. 2015). Although caution needs to be exerted when extrapolating results from animals to patients, this study highlights the power of this approach to link magnetic resonance imaging findings to their histopathological origins (Riga et al. 2014). 5-Methoxy-N,N-dimethyltryptamine is of potential interest for schizophrenia research owing to its hallucinogenic properties. Moreover, regional brain activity was assessed by BOLD fMRI. This, together with the reversal by antipsychotic drugs, suggests that the observed cortical alterations are related to the psychotomimetic action of 5-MeO-DMT. Overall, the present model may help to understand the neurobiological basis of hallucinations and to identify new targets in antipsychotic drug development (Vernon et al. 2014). Haloperidol, a dopamine D2/D3 receptor antagonist and placebo were administered to 25 smokers and 25 non-smoking controls in a double-blind randomized cross-over design while performing a Go/NoGo task during fMRI scanning. The current findings suggest that altered baseline dopamine levels in addicted individuals may contribute to the observed reduction in inhibitory control in these populations (Luijten et al. 2013). The findings identify possible systems underlying pathogenesis and treatment efficacy in disorders of dopamine deficiency (Cole et al. 2013). Haloperidol was associated with a significantly greater increase in regional cerebral blood flow in the left putamen and posterior cingulate, and a significantly greater decrease in regional cerebral blood flow in frontal regions compared to risperidone (Miller et al. 2001). fMRI study outlines the importance of further studies to investigate interindividual activation differences under different conditions especially focusing on basal ganglia (Müller et al. 2002). There was a significant increase in the T_1 value in the striate body 30 minutes and more (within two hours) after the administration of haloperidol (Fujimoto et al. 1987). fMRI recordings in which healthy volunteers were randomly assigned to one of three drug groups: amphetamine, haloperidol, and placebo (Diaconescu et al. 2010). fMRI is a non-invasive technique for brain mapping and mostly performed using changes of the BOLD signal. It has been widely used to investigate patients with schizophrenia (Röder et al. 2013). In schizophrenia and Parkinson's disease, cortical and subcortical motor organization is influenced by primary disease conditions and neuroleptic treatment (Müller et al. 2003). fMRI of the brain to demonstrate the efficacy of drug treatment inhibited both the subjective presence of phantoms and the fMRI brain activation initiated by these phantoms. These results demonstrate that phantom taste and smell can be revealed by fMRI brain activation (Tost et al. 2006; Henkin et al. 2000). Haloperidol subjects did not show PE related activity in any of these regions (Pine et al. 2010; Pleger et al. 2009; Menon et al. 2007). The structural changes of the functional pattern were described by the findings of fMRI (Neuner et al. 2013). fMRI was performed to assess the blood oxygenation level dependent response in the ventral striatum of schizophrenics medicated with typical neuroleptics (Schlagenhauf et al. 2008). In the study by Luijten, haloperidol was orally administered 4 h before each scanning session in a double blind randomized cross-over design (Luijten et al. 2012). fMRI to assess the blood oxygen level dependency response in the ventral striatum of medicated schizophrenics and healthy control subjects during reward anticipation (Juckel et al. 2006). fMRI demonstrated reduced frontal blood flow relative to global cerebral perfusion in schizophrenia patients. Overall, neuroimaging literature provides reliable evidence of frontal impairments in schizophrenia, although the average magnitude of difference between patients and controls is insufficient to defend a frontal lobe dysfunction hypo-thesis, as far as brain volume, resting cerebral metabolism or blood flow are concerned (Stip 2006). The normal response to somatosensory stimulation appears to be poised between two abnormal responses produced by two physiologically different types of seizures (Nersesyan et al. 2004). Haloperidol changed the habituation to the absolute pain intensity over time. More precisely, in the placebo condition, activity in left postcentral gyrus and midcingulate cortex increased linearly with pain intensity only in the beginning of the experiment and subsequently habituated (Bauch et al. 2017). Dopaminergic stimulation increased activation primarily in the posterior regions of the working memory network compared with dopaminergic blockade using a whole brain cluster-level corrected analysis. The dopaminergic medications did not affect working memory performance (Dumas, et al. 2017). fMRI blood oxygen level dependent signal has been studied in the context of antipsychotic treatment (Abbott, et al. 2013). Although the mechanisms of the antipsychotic properties are still not fully understood, new studies are warrented (Zuardi et al. 2012). fMRI replicated in larger studies may help unify and extend current hypotheses on dopaminergic dysfunction, salience processing and pathogenesis of delusions (Sarpal et al. 2016; Raij et al. 2015). Independent component analysis has identified temporally cohesive but spatially distributed neural networks (Abbott et al. 2011). Psychotic disorders are characterized by significant deficits in attentional control, but the neurobiological mechanisms underlying these deficits early in the course of illness prior to extensive pharmacotherapy are not well understood (Ikuta et al. 2014). Schizophrenia is characterized by an abnormal dopamine system, and dopamine blockade is the primary mechanism of antipsychotic treatment (Insel et al. 2014). fMRI has been increasingly used to investigate the neurobiology of schizophrenia by Röder and coworkers. This technique relies on changes in the blood-oxygen-level-dependent (BOLD) - signal, which changes in response to neural activity (Gu et al. 2014; Röder et al. 2010). These results suggest that schizophrenia is associated with more complex signal patterns when compared to healthy controls, supporting the increase in complexity hypothesis, where system complexity increases with age or disease, and also consistent with the notion that schizophrenia is characterised by a dysregulation of the nonlinear dynamics of underlying neuronal systems (Sokunbi et al. 2014; Machielsen et al. 2014). Pharmacological magnetic resonance imaging (phMRI) of the brain has become a widely used tool in both preclinical and clinical drug research (Bruns et al. 2015). However, little is known regarding the neuropsychological significance of resting state functional magnetic resonance imaging (rs-fMRI) activity early in the course of psychosis (Argyelan et al. 2015). Antipsychotic medications have established clinical benefit, but there are few neuroimaging studies before and after initiating antipsychotic medication to assess drug influence on brain circuitry. Attention and motor learning tasks are promising approaches for examining treatment-related changes in frontostriatal systems (Keedy et al. 2015; Kumari, et al. 2015). The neural mechanisms underlying this dysfunction remain unclear, with functional neuroimaging studies reporting increased, decreased or unchanged activation compared to controls (Ettinger et al. 2011). fMRI opens up new areas of research and a new approach for drug development, as it is an integrative tool to investigate entire networks within the brain (Hampel et al. 2011; Keedy et al. 2009; Nahas et al. 2003). fMRI has been used to examine the modulatory effects of acute psychopharmacological intervention on brain activation during four different cognitive tasks: overt verbal fluency, random movement generation, n-back and a spatial object memory task (Fusar-Poli et al. 2007). fMRI has been used to test whether depressed and manic bipolar disorder patients differ in terms of activity in cortical and subcortical brain areas and to examine the effects of psychotropic medication (Adragna 2012; Karch et al. 2012; Pavuluri et al. 2012; Caligiuri et al. 2003). Several studies have shown that patients with schizophrenia underactivate brain regions involved in theory of mind relative to controls during functional brain imaging (Brüne et al. 2008; Stip et al. 2005). Studies to examine patterns of cortical activation underlying D-cycloserine's therapeutic efficacy in schizophrenic patients using fMRI have also been performed (Pavuluri et al. 2010; Yurgelun-Todd et al. 2005).

CONCLUSION

The FMRI study investigated the effects of pharmacotherapy on brain function. Noninvasive detection of biomarkers allows for the dynamic evaluation of brain function.

ACKNOWLEDGMENTS

Dorota Bartusik-Aebisher acknowledges support from the National Center of Science NCN (New drug delivery systems-MRI study, Grant OPUS-13 number 2017/25/B/ST4/02481).

REFERENCES

Abbott, C. C., Jaramillo, A., Wilcox, C. E., Hamilton, D. A. (2013). Antipsychotic drug effects in schizophrenia: a review of longitudinal FMRI investigations and neural interpretations. *Current Medicinal Chemistry, 20*:428-37.

Abbott, C., Juárez, M., White, T., Gollub, R. L., Pearlson, G. D., Bustillo, J., Lauriello, J., Ho, B., Bockholt, H. J., Clark, V. P., Magnotta, V., Calhoun, V. D. (2011). Antipsychotic dose and diminished neural modulation: a multi-site fMRI study. *Progress in Neuro-Psychopharmacology & Biological Psychiatry, 35*:473-82.

Adragna, M. S. (2012). A functional magnetic resonance imaging study of risperidone and divalproex. *Journal of the American Academy of Child and Adolescent Psychiatry, 51*:652.

Argyelan, M., Gallego, J. A., Robinson, D. G., Ikuta, T., Sarpal, D., John, M., Kingsley, P. B., Kane, J., Malhotra, A. K., Szeszko, P. R. (2015). Abnormal resting state FMRI activity predicts processing speed deficits in first-episode psychosis. *Neuropsychopharmacology: Official Publication of the American College of Neuropsychopharmacology, 40*:1631-9.

Bauch, E. M., Andreou, C., Rausch, V. H., Bunzeck, N. (2017). Neural Habituation to Painful Stimuli Is Modulated by Dopamine: Evidence from a Pharmacological fMRI Study. *Frontiers in Human Neuroscience, 11*:630.

Bolstad I, Andreassen OA, Groote I, Server A, Sjaastad I, Kapur S, Jensen J (2015) Effects of haloperidol and aripiprazole on the human mesolimbic motivational system: A pharmacological fMRI study. *European Neuropsychopharmacology, 25*:2252-2261.

Bolstad, I., Andreassen, O. A., Groote, I. R., Haatveit, B., Server, A., Jensen, J. (2015). No difference in frontal cortical activity during an executive functioning task after acute doses of aripiprazole and haloperidol. *Frontiers in Human Neuroscience, 9*:296.

Brassen S, Tost H, Höhn F, Weber-Fahr W, Klein S, Braus DF (2016) Haloperidol challenge in healthy male humans: a functional magnetic resonance imaging study. *Neuroscience Letter,* 340:193-196.

Braus DF, Ende G, Weber-Fahr W, Sartorius A, Krier A, Hubrich-Ungureanu P, Ruf M, Stuck S, Henn FA (1999) Antipsychotic drug effects on motor activation measured by functional magnetic resonance imaging in schizophrenic patients. *Schizophrenia Research,* 39:19-29.

Brüne, M., Lissek, S., Fuchs, N., Witthaus, H., Peters, S., Nicolas, V., Juckel, G., Tegenthoff, M. (2008). An fMRI study of theory of mind in schizophrenic patients with "passivity" symptoms. *Neuropsychologia,* 46:1992-2001.

Bruns, A., Mueggler, T., Künnecke, B., Risterucci, C., Prinssen, E. P., Wettstein, J. G., von Kienlin, M. (2015). "Domain gauges": A reference system for multivariate profiling of brain fMRI activation patterns induced by psychoactive drugs in rats. *NeuroImage, 112*:70-85.

Caligiuri, M. P., Brown, G. G., Meloy, M. J., Eberson, S. C., Kindermann, S. S., Frank, L. R., Zorrilla, L. E., Lohr, J. B. (2003). An fMRI study of affective state and medication on cortical and subcortical brain regions during motor performance in bipolar disorder. *Psychiatry Research, 123*:171-82.

Cole DM, Beckmann CF, Oei NY, Both S, van Gerven JM, Rombouts SA (2013) Differential and distributed effects of dopamine neuromodulations on resting-state network connectivity. *Neuroimage,* 78:59-67.

Cole, D. M., Oei, N. Y., Soeter, R. P., Both, S., van Gerven, J. M., Rombouts, S. A., Beckmann, C. F. (2013). Dopamine-dependent architecture of cortico-subcortical network connectivity. *Cerebral Cortex, 23*:1509-16.

Diaconescu, A. O., Menon, M., Jensen, J., Kapur, S., McIntosh, A. R. (2010). Dopamine-induced changes in neural network patterns supporting aversive conditioning. *Brain Research, 1313*:143-61.

Dumas, J. A., Filippi, C. G., Newhouse, P. A., Naylor, M. R. (2017). Dopaminergic contributions to working memory-related brain activation in postmenopausal women. *Menopause: the Journal of the North American Menopause Society, 24*:163-170.

Ettinger, U., Williams, S. C., Fannon, D., Premkumar, P., Kuipers, E., Möller, H. J., Kumari, V. (2011). Functional magnetic resonance imaging of a parametric working memory task in schizophrenia: relationship with performance and effects of antipsychotic treatment. *Psychopharmacology, 216*:17-27.

Fujimoto, T., Nakano, T., Fujii, M., Okada, A,, Harada, K., Yokoyama, Y., Uchida, T., Tsuji, T., Igata, A., Asakura, T. (1987). Changes in proton T1 in dog brains due to the administration of haloperidol. *Magnetic Resonance Imaging, 5*:469-74.

Fusar-Poli, P., Broome, M. R., Matthiasson, P., Williams, S. C., Brammer, M., McGuire, P. K. (2007). Effects of acute antipsychotic treatment on brain activation in first episode psychosis: an fMRI study. *European Neuropsychopharmacology: the Journal of the European College of Neuropsychopharmacology, 17*:492-500.

Goozee R, O'Daly O, Handley R, Reis Marques T, Taylor H, McQueen G, Hubbard K, Pariante C, Mondelli V, Reinders AA, Dazzan P (2017) Effects of aripiprazole and haloperidol on neural activation during a simple motor task in healthy individuals: A functional MRI study. *Human Brain Mapping, 38:*1833-1845.

Goozee, R., Reinders, A. A. T. S., Handley, R., Marques, T., Taylor, H., O'Daly, O., McQueen, G., Hubbard, K., Mondelli, V., Pariante, C., Dazzan, P. (2016). Effects of aripiprazole and haloperidol on neural activation during the n-back in healthy individuals: A functional MRI study. *Schizophrenia research, 173*:174-181.

Gu, V., Mohamed Ali, O., L'Abbée Lacas, K., Debruille, J. B. (2014). Investigating the effects of antipsychotics and schizotypy on the N400 using event-related potentials and semantic categorization. *Journal of visualized experiments: JoVE, 93*:e52082.

Hampel, H., Prvulovic, D., Teipel, S. J., Bokde, A. L. (2011). Recent developments of functional magnetic resonance imaging research for drug development in Alzheimer's disease. *Progress in Neurobiology, 95*:570-8.

Hagino, H., Tabuchi, E., Kurachi, M., Saitoh, O., Sun, Y., Kondoh, T., Ono, T., Torii, K. (1998). Effects of D2 dopamine receptor agonist and antagonist on brain activity in the rat assessed by functional magnetic resonance imaging. *Brain Research*, *813*:367-73.

Hawkes, R. C., Holland, G. N., Moore, M. S. et al. (1980) Nuclear magnetic resonance tomography of the brain a preliminary clinicall assessment with demonstration of pathology. *Journal of Computed Assisted Tomography*, 4: 577-86.

Henkin, R. I., Levy, L. M., Lin, C. S. (2000). Taste and smell phantoms revealed by brain functional MRI (fMRI). *Journal of Computer Assisted Tomography*, *24*:106-23.

Insel, C., Reinen, J., Weber, J., Wager, T. D., Jarskog, L. F., Shohamy, D., Smith, E. E. (2014). Antipsychotic dose modulates behavioral and neural responses to feedback during reinforcement learning in schizophrenia. *Cognitive, Affective & Behavioral Neuroscience*, *14*:189-201.

Ikuta, T., Robinson, D. G., Gallego, J. A., Peters, B. D., Gruner, P., Kane, J., John, M., Sevy, S., Malhotra, A. K., Szeszko, P. R. (2014). Subcortical modulation of attentional control by second-generation antipsychotics in first-episode psychosis. *Psychiatry Research*, *221*:127-34.

Juckel, G., Schlagenhauf, F., Koslowski, M., Filonov, D., Wüstenberg, T., Villringer, A., Knutson, B., Kienast, T., Gallinat, J., Wrase, J., Heinz, A. (2006). Dysfunction of ventral striatal reward prediction in schizophrenic patients treated with typical, not atypical, neuroleptics. *Psychopharmacology*, *187*:222-8.

Karch, S., Pogarell, O., Mulert, C. (2012). Functional magnetic resonance imaging and treatment strategies in schizophrenia. *Current Pharmaceutical Biotechnology*, *13*:1622-9.

Keedy, S. K., Reilly, J. L., Bishop, J. R., Weiden, P. J., Sweeney, J. A. (2015). Impact of antipsychotic treatment on attention and motor learning systems in first-episode schizophrenia. *Schizophrenia Bulletin*, *41*:355-65.

Keedy, S. K., Rosen, C., Khine, T., Rajarethinam, R., Janicak, P. G., Sweeney, J. A. (2009). An fMRI study of visual attention and sensorimotor function before and after antipsychotic treatment in first-episode schizophrenia. *Psychiatry Research, 172*:16-23.

Kumari, V., Ettinger, U., Lee, S. E., Deuschl, C., Anilkumar, A. P., Schmechtig, A., Corr, P. J., Ffytche, D. H., Williams, S. C. (2015). Common and distinct neural effects of risperidone and olanzapine during procedural learning in schizophrenia: a randomised longitudinal fMRI study. *Psychopharmacology, 232*:3135-47.

Lahti AC, Weiler MA, Holcomb HH, Tamminga CA, Cropsey KL (2009) Modulation of limbic circuitry predicts treatment response to antipsychotic medication: a functional imaging study in schizophrenia. *Neuropsychopharmacology* 34:2675-2690.

Luijten, M., Veltman, D. J., Hester, R., Smits, M., Nijs, I. M., Pepplinkhuizen, L., Franken, I. H. (2013). The role of dopamine in inhibitory control in smokers and non-smokers: a pharmacological fMRI study. *European neuropsychopharmacology: the journal of the European College of Neuropsychopharmacology, 23*:1247-56.

Luijten, M., Veltman, D. J., Hester, R., Smits, M., Pepplinkhuizen, L., Franken, I. H. (2012). Brain activation associated with attentional bias in smokers is modulated by a dopamine antagonist. *Neuropsychopharmacology: official publication of the American College of Neuropsychopharmacology, 37*:2772-9.

Machielsen, M. W., Veltman, D. J., van den Brink, W., de Haan, L. (2014). The effect of clozapine and risperidone on attentional bias in patients with schizophrenia and a cannabis use disorder: An fMRI study. *Journal of psychopharmacology / British Association for Psychopharmacology, 28*:633-42.

Madularu, D., Kulkarni, P., Ferris, C. F., Brake, W. G. (2015). Changes in brain volume in response to estradiol levels, amphetamine sensitization and haloperidol treatment in awake female rats. *Brain Research, 1618*:100-10.

Menon, M., Jensen, J., Vitcu, I., Graff-Guerrero, A., Crawley, A., Smith, M. A., Kapur, S. (2007). Temporal difference modeling of the blood-oxygen level dependent response during aversive conditioning in humans: effects of dopaminergic modulation. *Biological Psychiatry*, *62*:765-72.

Müller, J. L., Klein, H. E. (2000). Neuroleptic therapy influences basal ganglia activation: a functional magnetic resonance imaging study comparing controls to haloperidol- and olanzapine-treated inpatients. *Psychiatry and Clinical Neurosciences, 54*:653-8.

Müller, J. L., Röder, C., Schuierer, G., Klein, H. E. (2002). Subcortical overactivation in untreated schizophrenic patients: a functional magnetic resonance image finger-tapping study. *Psychiatry and clinical Neurosciences, 56*:77-84.

Müller, J. L., Röder, C. H., Schuierer, G., Klein, H. (2002). Motor-induced brain activation in cortical, subcortical and cerebellar regions in schizophrenic inpatients. A whole brain fMRI fingertapping study. *Progress in Neuro-Psychopharmacology & Biological Psychiatry*, *26*:421-6.

Müller, J. L., Deuticke, C., Putzhammer, A., Röder, C. H., Hajak, G., Winkler, J. (2003). Schizophrenia and Parkinson's disease lead to equal motor-related changes in cortical and subcortical brain activation: an fMRI fingertapping study. *Psychiatry and Clinical Neurosciences, 57*:562-8.

Nahas, Z., George, M. S., Horner, M. D., Markowitz, J. S., Li, X., Lorberbaum, J. P., Owens, S. D., McGurk, S., DeVane, L., Risch, S. C. (2003). Augmenting atypical antipsychotics with a cognitive enhancer (donepezil) improves regional brain activity in schizophrenia patients: a pilot double-blind placebo controlled BOLD fMRI study. *Neurocase*, *9*:274-82.

Nersesyan, H., Herman, P., Erdogan, E., Hyder, F., Blumenfeld, H. (2004). Relative changes in cerebral blood flow and neuronal activity in local microdomains during generalized seizures. *Journal of Cerebral Blood Flow and Metabolism: Official Journal of the International Society of Cerebral Blood Flow and Metabolism, 24*:1057-68.

Neuner, I., Schneider, F., Shah, N. J. (2013). Functional neuroanatomy of tics. *International Review of Neurobiology, 112*:35-71.

Pavuluri, M. N., Passarotti, A. M., Fitzgerald, J. M., Wegbreit, E., Sweeney, J. A. (2012). Risperidone and divalproex differentially engage the fronto-striato-temporal circuitry in pediatric mania: a pharmacological functional magnetic resonance imaging study. *Journal of the American Academy of Child and Adolescent Psychiatry, 51*:157-170.

Pavuluri, M. N., Passarotti, A. M., Parnes, S. A., Fitzgerald, J. M., Sweeney, J. A. (2010). A pharmacological functional magnetic resonance imaging study probing the interface of cognitive and emotional brain systems in pediatric bipolar disorder. *Journal of Child and Adolescent Psychopharmacology, 20*:395-406.

Pine, A., Shiner, T., Seymour, B., Dolan, R. J. (2010). Dopamine, time, and impulsivity in humans. *The Journal of Neuroscience: the Official Journal of the Society for Neuroscience, 30*:8888-96.

Pleger, B., Ruff, C. C., Blankenburg, F., Klöppel, S., Driver, J., Dolan, R. J. (2009). Influence of dopaminergically mediated reward on somatosensory decision-making. *PLoS Biology, 7*:e1000164.

Raij, T. T., Mäntylä, T., Kieseppä, T., Suvisaari, J. (2015). Aberrant functioning of the putamen links delusions, antipsychotic drug dose, and compromised connectivity in first episode psychosis--Preliminary fMRI findings. *Psychiatry Research, 233*:201-11.

Riga, M. S., Soria, G., Tudela, R., Artigas, F., Celada, P. (2014). The natural hallucinogen 5-MeO-DMT, component of Ayahuasca, disrupts cortical function in rats: reversal by antipsychotic drugs. *The International Journal of Neuropsychopharmacology / Official Scientific Journal of the Collegium Internationale Neuropsycho-pharmacologicum (CINP), 17*:1269-82.

Röder, C. H., Dieleman, S., van der Veen, F. M., Linden, D. (2013). Systematic review of the influence of antipsychotics on the blood oxygenation level-dependent signal of functional magnetic resonance imaging. *Current Medicinal Chemistry, 20*:448-61.

Röder, C. H., Hoogendam, J. M., van der Veen, F. M. (2010). FMRI, antipsychotics and schizophrenia. Influence of different antipsychotics on BOLD-signal. *Current Pharmaceutical Design, 16*:2012-25.

Sarpal, D. K., Argyelan, M., Robinson, D. G., Szeszko, P. R., Karlsgodt, K. H., John, M., Weissman, N., Gallego, J. A., Kane, J. M., Lencz, T., Malhotra, A. K. (2016). Baseline Striatal Functional Connectivity as a Predictor of Response to Antipsychotic Drug Treatment. *The American Journal of Psychiatry*, *173*:69-77.

Schlagenhauf, F., Juckel, G., Koslowski, M., Kahnt, T., Knutson, B., Dembler, T., Kienast, T., Gallinat, J., Wrase, J., Heinz, A. (2008). Reward system activation in schizophrenic patients switched from typical neuroleptics to olanzapine. *Psychopharmacology*, *196*:673-84.

Sokunbi, M. O., Gradin, V. B., Waiter, G. D., Cameron, G. G., Ahearn, T. S., Murray, A. D., Steele, D. J., Staff, R. T. (2014). Nonlinear complexity analysis of brain FMRI signals in schizophrenia. *PloS one*, *9*:e95146.

Stip, E. (2006). Cognition, schizophrenia and the effect of antipsychotics. *Encephale*, *32*:341-50.

Stip, E., Fahim, C., Mancini-Marïe, A., Bentaleb, L. A., Mensour, B., Mendrek, A., Beauregard, M. (2005). Restoration of frontal activation during a treatment with quetiapine: an fMRI study of blunted affect in schizophrenia. *Progress in Neuro-Psychopharmacology & Biological Psychiatry*, *29*:21-6.

Tost, H., Meyer-Lindenberg, A., Klein, S., Schmitt, A., Höhn, F., Tenckhoff, A., Ruf, M., Ende, G., Rietschel, M., Henn, F. A., Braus, D. F. (2006). D2 antidopaminergic modulation of frontal lobe function in healthy human subjects. *Biological Psychiatry*, *60*:1196-205.

Vernon, A. C., Natesan, S., Crum, W. R., Cooper, J. D., Modo, M., Williams, S. C., Kapur, S. (2012). Contrasting effects of haloperidol and lithium on rodent brain structure: a magnetic resonance imaging study with postmortem confirmation. *Biological Psychiatry*, *71*:855-63.

Vernon, A. C., Crum, W. R., Lerch, J. P., Chege, W., Natesan, S., Modo, M., Cooper, J. D., Williams, S. C., Kapur, S. (2014). Reduced cortical volume and elevated astrocyte density in rats chronically treated with antipsychotic drugs-linking magnetic resonance imaging findings to cellular pathology. *Biological Psychiatry*, *75*:982-90.

Yurgelun-Todd, D. A., Coyle, J. T., Gruber, S. A., Renshaw, P. F., Silveri, M. M., Amico, E., Cohen, B., Goff, D. C. (2005). Functional magnetic resonance imaging studies of schizophrenic patients during word production: effects of D-cycloserine. *Psychiatry Research, 138*:23-31.

Zuardi, A. W., Crippa, J. A., Hallak, J. E., Bhattacharyya, S., Atakan, Z., Martin-Santos, R., McGuire, P. K., Guimarães, F. S. (2012). A critical review of the antipsychotic effects of cannabidiol: 30 years of a translational investigation. *Current Pharmaceutical Design, 18*:5131-40.

In: The Pharmacological Guide to Haloperidol   ISBN: 978-1-53614-700-1
Editor: Amor Harland   © 2019 Nova Science Publishers, Inc.

Chapter 6

APPLICATIONS OF ^{1}H AND ^{19}F MRI
TO MONITOR HALOPERIDOL

David Aebisher[*], *Dorota Bartusik-Aebisher*
and Łukasz Ożóg

Faculty of Medicine, University of Rzeszów,
Rzeszów, Poland

ABSTRACT

In this chapter we will provide a review of studies that have used
magnetic resonance imaging (MRI) to monitor haloperidol *in vivo*.
Applications of ^{1}H and ^{19}F MRI in drug monitoring will be discussed. A
presentation and list of recent studies using ^{19}F MRI for drug detection *in
vivo* will also be presented. Our objective in this chapter is to provide
reference information to the reader pertaining to the application of ^{1}H
MRI, ^{19}F MRI, and fMRI to haloperidol monitoring.

Keywords: fluorinated drug, haloperidol, ^{19}F MRI

[*] Corresponding Author Email: daebisher@ur.edu.pl.

INTRODUCTION

Haloperidol is widely used in the maintenance treatment of schizophrenia and other psychotic disorders, but knowledge concerning its pharmacokinetics at the injected region is very limited. Magnetic resonance imaging (MRI) studies suggest that antipsychotic-treated patients with schizophrenia show a decrease in gray-matter volumes (Vernon et al. 2012). Evaluating healthy individuals can allow investigation of the effects of different antipsychotics on cortical activation, independently of either disease-related pathology or previous treatment (Goozee et al. 2017). Functional magnetic resonance imaging (fMRI) was used to determine the acute blood oxygen level dependent effect (BOLD) of neuroleptic drugs in healthy male subjects' men (Brassen et al. 2016). In particular, fMRI measurements were obtained prior to as well as 1 h and 24 h after intravenous infusion of 5 mg haloperidol in six healthy young men (Brassen et al. 2016; Bartlett et al. 1991; Bartlett et al. 1944). Haloperidol is useful for this type of study because of its predominant antidopaminergic actions in the brain with potent D2 dopamine family receptor blockade (Tamminga and Holcomb 2001).

Brain function and laterality in schizophrenia were investigated using fMRI (Madularu et al. 2016; Braus et al. 1999; Holcomb et al. 1996). This supports the use of pharmacological fMRI to study antipsychotic properties in humans (Bolstad et al. 2015). Dopaminergic medications, used to treat neurochemical pathology and resultant symptoms in neuropsychiatric disorders, are of mixed efficacy and regularly associated with behavioral side effects (Cole et al. 2013; Handley et al. 2013; Lahti et al. 2003). In addition, in these regions, some patterns seen at weeks 1 and 6 were distinctive, indexing neuronal changes related to an early and consolidated stage of drug response (Lahti et al. 2009; Lahti et al. 2005; Lahti et al. 2004). Haloperidol increased striatal metabolic rate more than olanzapine (Buchsbaum et al. 2007). Haloperidol was associated with a significantly greater increase in regional cerebral blood flow (Miller et al. 2001).

Patients on chronic haloperidol showed increased activity in the motor cortex and cerebellum (Molina et al. 2003; Sassa et al. 2002).

^{19}F magnetic resonance imaging MRI data suggest that *in vivo* ^{19}F MRI of fluorinated agents is possible and could have clinical and research applications in the neurosciences (Arndt et al. 1988). Fluorinated psychopharmacological agents were measured with fluorine-19 nuclear magnetic resonance spectroscopy in the brain of intact rats that had been treated with fluphenazine (Bartels et al. 1986). *In vivo* ^{19}F-NMR spectroscopy measurements of trifluorinated neuroleptics were made in rat brain as well as in the human brain (Bartels et al. 1991). Fluorine-19 NMR spectroscopy was used to monitor the anti-depressant drug fluoxetine (and its metabolite norfluoxetine) *in vivo* in the human brain. The *in vivo* signal arose about equally from fluoxetine and the active metabolite norfluoxetine, as demonstrated by the *in vitro* ^{19}F NMR spectrum of the lipophilic extract of a small section of brain (Komoroski et al. 1994). *In vivo* ^{19}F resonance spectroscopy measurements of trifluorinated neuroleptics and later trifluorinated antidepressants began with animal experiments in 1983. The extension of the animal studies to humans might facilitate a better treatment of schizophrenic and depressive patients (Bartels and Albert 1995). Results have demonstrated that the ^{19}F NMR method can be usefully applied to the determination of partition coefficients of many drugs having fluorine atoms without any separation procedure, especially for drugs which do not have absorption in the ultraviolet or visible region (Omran et al. 2002).

Reduced brain N-acetyl-aspartate (NAA) has been repeatedly found in chronic schizophrenia and suggests neuronal loss or dysfunction. Early in the illness, schizophrenia patients already demonstrate subtle reductions in NAA. Treatment with typical or atypical antipsychotic medications for several months does not result in NAA changes (Bustillo et al. 2008). N-acetylaspartate is present in high concentrations in the CNS and is found primarily in neurons. NAA is considered to be a marker of neuronal viability. Numerous magnetic resonance spectroscopy and postmortem studies have shown reductions of NAA in different brain regions in schizophrenia (Harte et al. 2005). Proton magnetic resonance spectroscopy studies of schizophrenic patients generally reveal reduced levels of N-acetyl aspartate when compared with healthy controls. Whether this reduction is due to the disease or to the drugs used for treatment remains an open question (Lindquist et al. 2011). Haloperidol is a ligand that can target sigma 2 receptors over-expressed in non-small cell lung cancer (Varshosaz et al. 2015). ^{1}H-MRS studies of schizophrenia suggest an effect of the disease or of antipsychotic medications on brain N-acetyl aspartate (NAA), a marker of neuronal viability (Bustillo et al. 2006). The pathogenesis of antipsychotic-induced disturbances of glucose homeostasis is still unclear. Increased visceral adiposity has been suggested to be a possible mediating mechanism (Mondelli et al. 2013; Roiz-Santiáñez et al. 2012; Buchsbaum et al. 2009). Caudate and hippocampal volume differences in patients with schizophrenia are associated with disease and antipsychotic treatment, but local shape alterations have not been thoroughly examined (Crum et al. 2016; McClure et al. 2013). Although caution needs to be exerted when extrapolating results from animals to patients, this study highlights the power of this approach to link magnetic resonance imaging findings to their histopathological origins (Vernon et al. 2014; Steiner et al. 2011). Literature review suggested a syndrome with a triad of symptoms: non-ketotic hyperglycemia, hemichorea, and T_1 MRI striatal hyperintensities. Patients have been presented who had a sustained therapeutic result from haloperidol and clonazepam (Al-Quliti et al. 2016). It is not known whether the magnitude of the structural brain abnormalities that underlie schizophrenia is a determinant of the extent to which patients respond to antipsychotic medication (Zipursky et al. 1998; Fujimoto et al. 1987). Patients with larger brain volumes may be more likely to experience the benefits of clozapine treatment and experience a subsequent worsening of their symptoms when treated with haloperidol (Arango et al. 2003).

Results have shown that risperidone and haloperidol have significantly different effects on brain function, which may be related to their differences in efficacy and side effects. These findings emphasize the importance of controlling for both medication status and the individual antipsychotic in neuroimaging studies (Miller et al. 2001). Haloperidol treated patients exhibited significant decreases in gray matter volume (Lieberman et al. 2005; Halene et al. 2016). T_2 gradient sequences showed a peripheral rim of decreased signal intensity, which is the hemosiderin ring (Kongsakorn and Maroongroge 2015). MRI findings of four hemiballism cases have been described, and pathophysiology, pathogenesis and treatment of hemiballism were discussed (Vernon et al. 2011; Konagaya et al. 1990). Using time-lapse maps, the dynamics of schizophrenia progression, revealing spreading cortical changes that depend on the type of antipsychotic treatment was studied (Thompson et al. 2009). The cortical gray expansion may be relevant to the reported enhanced neurocognition and quality of life associated with SGA treatment (Garver et al. 2005). Regarding drug dosages, haloperidol has an advantage over flunitrazepam as a first infusion in safety (Hatta et al. 2010). The comorbidity of the two illnesses worsens clinical and therapeutic prognosis and also suggests interesting pathophysiological hypotheses (Canellas-Dols et al. 2017). Exposure to haloperidol-like drugs may in part account for the frontal NAA reductions previously reported in schizophrenia (Bustillo et al. 2001). Quantitative measures of T_1 and regional blood flow of the healthy human brain was measured after received olanzapine (7.5 mg), haloperidol (3 mg), or placebo (Hawkins et al. 2018). The data of others demonstrate the possibility of obtaining *in vivo* pharmacokinetics of fluorinated agents in the rat brain. ^{19}F NMR is expected to become an important tool in neurochemical research (Albert et al. 1990; Yanagisawa et al. 2017). ^{19}F nuclear magnetic resonance was used as a suitable analytical tool for the identification and selective determination of haloperidol in human serum and pharmaceutical preparations (Shamsipur et al. 2007). Table 1 summarizes some important *in vivo* studies of haloperidol in animals and humans.

Table 1. Applications of Haloperidol

Reference	Dose of haloperidol	Purpose of the study	Test method/ technique	Animals or Humans
Bartels et al. 1986	-	noninvasive technique for determining fluorinated neuroleptics in live mammals	^{19}F MRS	rats
Fujimoto et al. 1987	singlet dose 20 mg	T1 time changes in dog brains due to the administration of haloperidol	^{1}H MRI	mongrel dogs
Bartlett et al. 1994	single dose 5 mg	brain's metabolic response	PET, fluorodeoxyglucose (FDG)	healthy humans
Zipursky et al. 1998	2-20 mg/day	magnitude of the structural brain abnormalities caused by drug treatment	^{1}H MRI	patients with first-episode psychosis
Braus et al. 1999	about 4 mg	drug effects on motor activation	fMRI	schizophrenic patients
Tamminga et al. 2001	0.3 mg/kg per day for 4 weeks	effect of reduced brain activity	PET, FDG	schizophrenic patients
Miller et al. 2001	11.2 ± 5.0 mg/day	effect on rCBF changes and to effects of drug on brain function	PET with ^{15}O water	schizophrenic patients
Miller et al. 2001	3-20 mg/day for 3 weeks	effects of drug on rCBF	PET with ^{15}O water and MRI	schizophrenic patients
Bustillo et al. 2001	-	effect on concentration of metabolites in the caudate nuclei and the left frontal lobe	^{1}H MRS	schizophrenic patients
Sassa et al. 2002	15 mg	diachronic change at the injection point and visualize its local distribution after intramuscular injection	^{19}F MRS and chemical shift imaging (CSI)	schizophrenic patients
Lahti et al. 2003	0.3 mg/kg for at least 4 weeks	identifying brain regions where drugs shows similar and dissimilar patterns of rCBF changes	PET with ^{15}O water	schizophrenic patients
Molina et al. 2003	5 mg/day for 2 days or 10-15 mg/day for 4 weeks	assessment the metabolic changes associated with treatment	FDG-PET	schizophrenic patients

Reference	Dose of haloperidol	Purpose of the study	Test method/ technique	Animals or Humans
Arango et al. 2003	20 mg/day for 4 weeks or 10-30 mg/day for 2 weeks	assessment the brain structure volume caused by drug treatment	^1H MRI	schizophrenic patients
Lahti et al. 2004	0.3 mg/kg for at least 4 weeks or 12 ± 4.5 mg/day for 12 ± 10 weeks	effects on rCBF changes	PET with ^{15}O water	schizophrenic patients and healthy normal volunteers
Lahti et al. 2005	singlet dose 10 mg	assessment the time course of functional brain changes and the rCBF changes	PET with ^{15}O water	medically healthy persons with schizophrenia
Lieberman et al. 2005	2-20 mg/day	assessment brain volume changes caused by drug treatment	^1H MRI	patients with first-episode psychosis
Garver et al. 2005	7 mg/day for 4 weeks	effects of drugs on cortical gray volumes	^1H MRI	schizophrenic patients
Harte et al. 2005	28.5 mg/kg/3 weeks for 24 weeks	effect on concentration of NAA in brain tissue	^1H MRS	rats
Bustillo et al. 2006	38 mg/kg/month for 6 months	effect of haloperidol on NAA, glutamate, and glutamine in several brain regions	^1H MRS	rats
Buchsbaum et al. 2007	20 mg/day for 8-9 weeks	assessment of brain activity and relative metabolic rates	PET with 18-F-deoxyglucose (FDG-PET) and anatomical MRI	medicated psychotic adolescents
Shamsipur et al. 2007	60-600 µg/ml	identification and selective determination of haloperidol in human serum	^{19}F NMR	human serum
Bustillo et al. 2008	2-12 mg/day for 2 years	effect on concentration of metabolites in the frontal and occipital lobes, caudate nucleus, and cerebellum	^1H MRS	schizophrenic patients and healthy humans
Lahti et al. 2009	10 mg for 6 days or 10-20 mg for 5 weeks	effects on rCBF changes in the brain due to treatment	PET with ^{15}O water	schizophrenic patients

Table 1. (Continued)

Reference	Dose of haloperidol	Purpose of the study	Test method/ technique	Animals or Humans
Buchsbaum et al. 2009	4-16 mg/day for 6 weeks	assessment the difference of frontal lobe metabolism in patients treated to examine the differences in regional effects of drugs	FDG-PET and MRI	schizophrenic patients
Thompson et al. 2009	2-20 mg/day for 16 weeks	spreading cortical changes caused by drug treatment	^{1}H MRI	schizophrenic patients
Vernon et al. 2011	2 mg/kg/day for 8 weeks	effect of chronic antipsychotic treatment on brain structure	^{1}H MRI	rats
Lindquist et al. 2011	0.2-2 mg/kg/day for 6 months	effect of long term antipsychotic treatment on metabolite concentrations in rat striatum	^{1}H MRS	rats
Vernon et al. 2012	0.5 mg/kg/day or 2 mg/kg/day	effects on brain volume	^{1}H MRI	rats
Roiz-Santiáñez et al. 2012	3-9 mg/day for 1 year	effects of low doses of haloperidol on brain cortical thickness	^{1}H MRI	schizophrenic patients
Cole et al. 2013	singlet dose 3 mg	effect on large-scale resting-state network connectivity relationships in the healthy human brain	fMRI	healthy humans
Handley et al. 2013	singlet dose 3 mg	effect on resting cerebral blood flow (rCBF) in the human brain	^{1}H MRI	healthy humans
Mondelli et al. 2013	2 mg/kg/day for 8 weeks	effects of haloperidol on visceral fat deposition and on critical nodes of the insulin signaling pathway	^{1}H MRI	rats
McClure et al. 2013	2-20 mg/day for 47 months	localized differences in caudate and hippocampal shape caused by drug treatment	^{1}H MRI	schizophrenic patients
Vernon et al. 2014	2 mg/kg/day for 8 weeks	effect on brain structure, particularly the cerebral cortex	^{1}H MRI	rats
Bolstad et al. 2015	single dose 2 mg or 3 mg	effects on the human mesolimbic motivational system	fMRI	healthy humans

Reference	Dose of haloperidol	Purpose of the study	Test method/ technique	Animals or Humans
Brassen et al. 2016	single dose 5 mg/70 kg	cerebral psychopharmacological effects	fMRI	healthy humans
Madularu et al. 2016	0.25 mg/kg/day	increased BOLD activity in regions of interest and neural networks associated with schizophrenia	fMRI	rats
Crum et al. 2016	2 mg/kg/day for 8 weeks	effect of clinically relevant doses of either haloperidol on adult rat hippocampal volume	1H MRI; tensor-based morphometry (TBM)	rats
Halene et al. 2016	4 mg/kg/day for 6 months	assessment changes frontal gray and white matter volumes before and after of drug treatment	^1H MRI	macaque monkeys
Goozee et al. 2017	single dose 3 mg	motor function effects	fMRI	healthy humans
Yanagisawa et al. 2017	6-10 mg/kg	finding a potent ^{19}F MRI probe to evaluate dopaminergic presynaptic function in the striatum	^{19}F MRI; ^{19}F NMR	rats
Hawkins et al. 2018	singlet dose 3 mg	effect of a single clinically relevant dose of antipsychotics on CBF and qualitative T_1 measures of the brain	^1H MRI	healthy humans

CONCLUSION

In this chapter we provide new information to the reader about the potential for applying ^{19}F MRI, and ^1H MRI to haloperidol monitoring.

ACKNOWLEDGMENTS

Dorota Bartusik-Aebisher acknowledges support from the National Center of Science NCN (New drug delivery systems-MRI study, Grant OPUS-13 number 2017/25/B/ST4/02481).

REFERENCES

Albert, K., Rembold, H., Kruppa, G., Bayer, E., Bartels, M., Schmalzing, G. (1990). *In vivo* 19F nuclear magnetic resonance spectroscopy of trifluorinated neuroleptics in the rat. *NMR in Biomedicine*, 3(3):120-3.

Al-Quliti, K. W. and Assaedi, E. S. (2016). Hemichorea with unilateral MRI striatal hyperintensity in a Saudi patient with diabetes. *Neurosciences: The Official Journal of The Pan Arab Union of Neurological Sciences*, 21(1):56-9.

Arango, C., Breier, A., McMahon, R., Carpenter, W. T. Jr., Buchanan, R. W. (2003). The relationship of clozapine and haloperidol treatment response to prefrontal, hippocampal, and caudate brain volumes. *The American Journal of Psychiatry*, 160(8):1421-7.

Arndt, D. C., Ratner, A. V., Faull, K. F., Barchas, J. D., Young, S. W. (1988). 19F magnetic resonance imaging and spectroscopy of a fluorinated neuroleptic ligand: *in vivo* and *in vitro* studies. *Psychiatry Research*, 25(1):73-9.

Bartels, M. and Albert, K. (1995). Detection of psychoactive drugs using 19F MR spectroscopy. *Journal of Neural Transmission. General Section*, 99(1-3):1-6.

Bartels, M., Albert, K., Kruppa, G., Mann, K., Schroth, G., Tabarelli, S., Zabel, M. (1986). Fluorinated psychopharmacological agents: noninvasive observation by fluorine-19 nuclear magnetic resonance. *Psychiatry Research*, 18(3):197-201.

Bartels, M., Günther, U., Albert, K., Mann, K., Schuff, N., Stuckstedte, H. (1991). 19F nuclear magnetic resonance spectroscopy of neuroleptics: the first *in vivo* pharmacokinetics of trifluoperazine in the rat brain and the first *in vivo* spectrum of fluphenazine in the human brain. *Biological Psychiatry*, 30(7):656-62.

Bartlett, E. J., Brodie, J. D., Simkowitz, P., Dewey, S. L., Rusinek, H., Wolf, A. P., Fowler, J. S., Volkow, N. D., Smith, G., Wolkin, A. (1994). Effects of haloperidol challenge on regional cerebral glucose utilization in normal human subjects. *The American Journal of Psychiatry*, 151(5):681-86.

Bartlett, E. J., Wolkin, A., Brodie, J. D., Laska, E. M., Wolf, A. P., Sanfilipo, M. (1991). Importance of pharmacologic control in PET studies: effects of thiothixene and haloperidol on cerebral glucose utilization in chronic schizophrenia. *Psychiatry Research*, 40(2):115-24.

Bolstad, I., Andreassen, O. A., Groote, I., Server, A., Sjaastad, I., Kapur, S., Jensen, J. (2015). Effects of haloperidol and aripiprazole on the human mesolimbic motivational system: A pharmacological fMRI study. *European Neuropsychopharmacology: The Journal of The European College of Neuropsychopharmacology*, 25(12):2252-61.

Brassen, S., Tost, H., Höhn, F., Weber-Fahr, W., Klein, S., Braus, D. F. (2016). Haloperidol challenge in healthy male humans: a functional magnetic resonance imaging study. *Neuroscience Letters*, 340(3):193-96.

Braus, D. F., Ende, G., Weber-Fahr, W., Sartorius, A., Krier, A., Hubrich-Ungureanu, P., Ruf, M., Stuck, S., Henn, F. A. (1991). Antipsychotic drug effects on motor activation measured by functional magnetic resonance imaging in schizophrenic patients. *Schizophrenia Research*, 39(1):19-29.

Buchsbaum, M. S., Haznedar, M. M., Aronowitz, J., Brickman, A. M., Newmark, R. E., Bloom, R., Brand, J., Goldstein, K. E., Heath, D., Starson, M., Hazlett, E. A. (2007). FDG-PET in never-previously medicated psychotic adolescents treated with olanzapine or haloperidol. *Schizophrenia Research*, 94(1-3):293-305.

Buchsbaum, M. S., Haznedar, M., Newmark, R. E., Chu, K. W., Dusi, N., Entis, J. J., Goldstein, K. E., Goodman, C. R., Gupta, A., Hazlett, E., Iannuzzi, J., Torosjan, Y., Zhang, J., Wolkin, A. (2009). FDG-PET and MRI imaging of the effects of sertindole and haloperidol in the prefrontal lobe in schizophrenia. *Schizophrenia Research*, 114(1-3):161-71.

Bustillo, J. R., Lauriello, J., Rowland, L. M., Jung, R. E., Petropoulos, H., Hart, B. L., Blanchard, J., Keith, S. J., Brooks, W. M. (2001). Effects of chronic haloperidol and clozapine treatments on frontal and caudate neurochemistry in schizophrenia. *Psychiatry Research*, 107(3):135-49.

Bustillo, J. R., Rowland, L. M., Jung, R., Brooks, W. M., Qualls, C., Hammond, R., Hart, B., Lauriello, J. (2008). Proton magnetic resonance spectroscopy during initial treatment with antipsychotic medication in schizophrenia. *Neuropsychopharmacology: Official Publication of the American College of Neuropsychopharmacology*, 33(10):2456-66.

Bustillo, J., Barrow, R., Paz, R., Tang, J., Seraji-Bozorgzad, N., Moore, G. J., Bolognani, F., Lauriello, J., Perrone-Bizzozero, N., Galloway, M. P. (2006). Long-term treatment of rats with haloperidol: lack of an effect on brain N-acetyl aspartate levels. *Neuropsychopharmacology: Official Publication of The American College of Neuropsychopharmacology*, 31(4):751-6.

Canellas-Dols, F., Delgado, C., Arango-Lopez, C., Peraita-Adrados, R. (2017). Narcolepsy-cataplexy and psychosis: a case study. *Revista de Neurologia*, 65(2):70-74.

Cole, D. M., Beckmann, C. F., Oei, N. Y., Both, S., van Gerven, J. M., Rombouts, S. A. (2013). Differential and distributed effects of dopamine neuromodulations on resting-state network connectivity. *NeuroImage*, 78:59-67.

Crum, W. R., Danckaers, F., Huysmans, T., Cotel, M. C., Natesan, S., Modo, M. M., Sijbers, J., Williams, S. C., Kapur, S., Vernon, A. C. (2016). Chronic exposure to haloperidol and olanzapine leads to common and divergent shape changes in the rat hippocampus in the absence of grey-matter volume loss. *Psychological Medicine*, 46(15):3081-93.

Fujimoto, T., Nakano, T., Fujii, M., Okada, A., Harada, K., Yokoyama, Y., Uchida, T., Tsuji, T., Igata, A., Asakura, T. (1987). Changes in proton T1 in dog brains due to the administration of haloperidol. *Magnetic Resonance Imaging*, 5(6):469-74.

Garver, D. L., Holcomb, J. A., Christensen, J. D. (2005). Cerebral cortical gray expansion associated with two second-generation antipsychotics. *Biological Psychiatry*, 58(1):62-6.

Goozee, R., O'Daly, O., Handley, R., Reis Marques, T., Taylor, H., McQueen, G., Hubbard, K., Pariante, C., Mondelli, V., Reinders, A.

A., Dazzan, P. (2017). Effects of aripiprazole and haloperidol on neural activation during a simple motor task in healthy individuals: A functional MRI study. *Human Brain Mapping*, 38(4):1833-45.

Halene, T. B., Kozlenkov, A., Jiang, Y., Mitchell, A. C., Javidfar, B., Dincer, A., Park, R., Wiseman, J., Croxson, P. L., Giannaris, E. L., Hof, P. R., Roussos, P., Dracheva, S., Hemby, S, E., Akbarian, S. (2016). NeuN+ neuronal nuclei in non-human primate prefrontal cortex and subcortical white matter after clozapine exposure. *Schizophrenia Research*, 170(2-3):235-44.

Handley, R., Zelaya, F. O., Reinders, A. A., Marques, T. R., Mehta, M. A., O'Gorman, R., Alsop, D. C., Taylor, H., Johnston, A., Williams, S., McGuire, P., Pariante, C. M., Kapur, S., Dazzan, P. (2013). Acute effects of single-dose aripiprazole and haloperidol on resting cerebral blood flow (rCBF) in the human brain. *Human Brain Mapping*, 34(2):272-82.

Harte, M. K., Bachus, S. B., Reynolds, G. P. (2005). Increased N-acetylaspartate in rat striatum following long-term administration of haloperidol. *Schizophrenia Research*, 75(2-3):303-8.

Hatta, K., Nakamura, M., Yoshida, K., Hamakawa, H., Wakejima, T., Nishimura, T., Furuta, K., Kawabata, T., Hirata, T., Usui, C., Nakamura, H., Sawa, Y. (2010). A prospective naturalistic multicentre study of intravenous medications in behavioural emergencies: haloperidol versus flunitrazepam. *Psychiatry Research*, 178(1):182-5.

Hawkins, P. C. T., Wood, T. C., Vernon, A. C., Bertolino, A., Sambataro, F., Dukart, J., Merlo-Pich, E., Risterucci, C., Silber-Baumann, H., Walsh, E., Mazibuko, N., Zelaya, F. O., Mehta, M. A. (2018). An investigation of regional cerebral blood flow and tissue structure changes after acute administration of antipsychotics in healthy male volunteers. *Human Brain Mapping*, 39(1):319-331.

Holcomb, H. H., Cascella, N. G., Thaker, G. K., Medoff, D. R., Dannals, R. F., Tamminga, C. A. (1996). Functional sites of neuroleptic drug action in the human brain: PET/FDG studies with and without haloperidol. *The American Journal of Psychiatry*, 153(1):41-9.

116   *David Aebisher, Dorota Bartusik-Aebisher and Łukasz Ożóg*

Komoroski, R. A., Newton, J. E., Cardwell, D., Sprigg, J., Pearce, J., Karson, C. N. (1994). *In vivo* 19F spin relaxation and localized spectroscopy of fluoxetine in human brain. *Magnetic Resonance in Medicine*, 31(2):204-11.

Konagaya, M., Nakamuro, T., Sugata, T., Funakawa, I., Takayanagi, T. (1990). MRI study of hemiballism. *Clinical Neurology Rinsho Shinkeigaku*, 30(1):17-23.

Kongsakorn, N. and Maroongroge, P. (2015). A case of hemichorea caused by cerebral cavernous angioma. *Journal of the Medical Association of Thailand*, 98(9):165-9.

Lahti, A. C., Holcomb, H. H., Weiler, M. A., Medoff, D. R., Frey, K. N., Hardin, M., Tamminga, C. A. (2004). Clozapine but not haloperidol Re-establishes normal task-activated rCBF patterns in schizophrenia within the anterior cingulate cortex. *Neuropsychopharmacology: Official Publication of the American College of Neuropsychopharmacology*, 29(1):171-8.

Lahti, A. C., Holcomb, H. H., Weiler, M. A., Medoff, D. R., Tamminga, C. A. (2003). Functional effects of antipsychotic drugs: comparing clozapine with haloperidol. *Biological Psychiatry*, 53(7):601-8.

Lahti, A. C., Weiler, M. A., Holcomb, H. H., Tamminga, C. A., Cropsey, K. L. (2009). Modulation of limbic circuitry predicts treatment response to antipsychotic medication: a functional imaging study in schizophrenia. *Neuropsychopharmacology: Official Publication of the American College of Neuropsychopharmacology*, 34(13):2675-90.

Lahti, A. C., Weiler, M. A., Medoff, D. R., Tamminga, C. A., Holcomb, H. H. (2005). Functional effects of single dose first- and second-generation antipsychotic administration in subjects with schizophrenia. *Psychiatry Research*, 139(1):19-30.

Lieberman, J. A., Tollefson, G. D., Charles, C., Zipursky, R., Sharma, T., Kahn, R. S., Keefe, R. S., Green, A. I., Gur, R. E., McEvoy, J., Perkins, D., Hamer, R. M., Gu, H., Tohen, M.; HGDH Study Group. (2005). Antipsychotic drug effects on brain morphology in first-episode psychosis. *Archives of General Psychiatry*, 62(4):361-70.

Lindquist, D. M., Dunn, R. S., Cecil, K. M. (2011). Long term antipsychotic treatment does not alter metabolite concentrations in rat striatum: an *in vivo* magnetic resonance spectroscopy study. *Schizophrenia Research*, 128(1-3):83-90.

Madularu, D., Kulkarni, P., Yee, J. R., Kenkel, W. M., Shams, W. M., Ferris, C. F., Brake, W. G. (2016). High estrogen and chronic haloperidol lead to greater amphetamine-induced BOLD activation in awake, amphetamine-sensitized female rats. *Hormones and Behavior*, 82:56-63.

McClure, R. K., Styner, M., Maltbie, E., Lieberman, J. A., Gouttard, S., Gerig, G., Shi, X., Zhu, H. (2013). Localized differences in caudate and hippocampal shape are associated with schizophrenia but not antipsychotic type. *Psychiatry Research*, 211(1):1-10.

Miller, D. D., Andreasen, N. C., O'Leary, D. S., Watkins, G. L., Boles Ponto, L. L., Hichwa, R. D. (2001). Comparison of the effects of risperidone and haloperidol on regional cerebral blood flow in schizophrenia. *Biological Psychiatry*, 49(8):704-15.

Miller, D. D., Andreasen, N. C., O'Leary, D. S., Watkins, G. L., Boles Ponto, L. L., Hichwa, R. D. (2001). Comparison of the effects of risperidone and haloperidol on regional cerebral blood flow in schizophrenia. *Biological Psychiatry*, 49(8):704-15.

Molina, V., Gispert, J. D., Reig, S., Sanz, J., Pascau, J., Santos, A., Palomo, T., Desco, M. (2003). Cerebral metabolism and risperidone treatment in schizophrenia. *Schizophrenia Research*, 60(1):1-7.

Mondelli, V., Anacker, C., Vernon, A. C., Cattaneo, A., Natesan, S., Modo, M., Dazzan, P., Kapur, S., Pariante, C. M. (2013). Haloperidol and olanzapine mediate metabolic abnormalities through different molecular pathways. *Translational Psychiatry*, 3:e208.

Omran, A. A., Kitamura, K., Takegami, S., Kume, M., Yoshida, M., El-Sayed, A. A., Mohamed, M. H., Abdel-Mottaleb, M. (2002). 19F NMR spectrometric determination of the partition coefficients of some fluorinated psychotropic drugs between phosphatidylcholine bilayer vesicles and water. *Journal of Pharmaceutical and Biomedical Analysis*, 30(4):1087-92.

Roiz-Santiáñez, R., Tordesillas-Gutiérrez, D., Ortíz-García de la Foz, V., Ayesa-Arriola, R., Gutiérrez, A., Tabarés-Seisdedos, R., Vázquez-Barquero, J. L., Crespo-Facorro, B. (2012). Effect of antipsychotic drugs on cortical thickness. A randomized controlled one-year follow-up study of haloperidol, risperidone and olanzapine. *Schizophrenia Research*, 141(1):22-8.

Sassa, T., Suhara, T., Ikehira, H., Obata, T., Girard, F., Tanada, S., Okubo, Y. (2002). 19F-magnetic resonance spectroscopy and chemical shift imaging for schizophrenic patients using haloperidol decanoate. *Psychiatry and Clinical Neurosciences*, 56(6):637-42.

Shamsipur, M., Shafiee-Dastgerdi, L., Talebpour, Z., Haghgoo, S. (2007). 19F NMR as a powerful technique for the assay of anti-psychotic drug haloperidol in human serum and pharmaceutical formulations. *Journal of Pharmaceutical and Biomedical Analysis*, 43(3):1116-21.

Steiner, J., Sarnyai, Z., Westphal, S., Gos, T., Bernstein, H. G., Bogerts, B., Keilhoff, G. (2011). Protective effects of haloperidol and clozapine on energy-deprived OLN-93 oligodendrocytes. *European Archives of Psychiatry and Clinical Neuroscience*, 261(7):477-82.

Tamminga, C., Holcomb, H. (2001). Neural networks: neural systems vi: basal ganglia. *The American Journal of Psychiatry*, 158(2):185.

Thompson, P. M., Bartzokis, G., Hayashi, K. M., Klunder, A. D., Lu, P. H., Edwards, N., Hong, M. S., Yu, M., Geaga, J. A., Toga, A. W., Charles, C., Perkins, D. O., McEvoy, J., Hamer, R. M., Tohen, M., Tollefson, G. D., Lieberman, J. A.; HGDH Study Group. (2009). Time-lapse mapping of cortical changes in schizophrenia with different treatments. *Cerebral Cortex*, 19(5):1107-23.

Varshosaz, J., Hassanzadeh, F., Mardani, A., Rostami, M. (2015). Feasibility of haloperidol-anchored albumin nanoparticles loaded with doxorubicin as dry powder inhaler for pulmonary delivery. *Pharmaceutical Development and Technology*, 20(2):183-96.

Vernon, A. C., Crum, W. R., Lerch, J. P., Chege, W., Natesan, S., Modo, M., Cooper, J. D., Williams, S. C., Kapur, S. (2014). Reduced cortical volume and elevated astrocyte density in rats chronically treated with antipsychotic drugs-linking magnetic resonance imaging findings to cellular pathology. *Biological Psychiatry*, 75(12):982-90.

Vernon, A. C., Natesan, S., Crum, W. R., Cooper, J. D., Modo, M., Williams, S. C., Kapur, S. (2012). Contrasting effects of haloperidol and lithium on rodent brain structure: a magnetic resonance imaging study with postmortem confirmation. *Biological Psychiatry*, 71(10):855-63.

Vernon, A. C., Natesan, S., Modo, M., Kapur, S. (2011). Effect of chronic antipsychotic treatment on brain structure: a serial magnetic resonance imaging study with ex vivo and postmortem confirmation. *Biological Psychiatry*, 69(10):936-44.

Yanagisawa, D., Oda, K., Inden, M., Morikawa, S., Inubushi, T., Taniguchi, T., Hijioka, M., Kitamura, Y., Tooyama, I. (2017). Fluorodopa is a promising Fluorine-19 MRI probe for evaluating striatal dopaminergic function in a rat model of Parkinson's disease. *Journal of Neuroscience Research*, 95(7):1485-94.

Zipursky, R. B., Zhang-Wong, J., Lambe, E. K., Bean, G., Beiser, M. (1998). MRI correlates of treatment response in first episode psychosis. *Schizophrenia Research*, 30(1):81-90.

INDEX

Duloxetine: Clinical Uses, Mechanism of Action and Efficacy

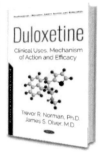

Authors: Trevor Norman, Ph.D. (University of Melbourne, Austin Hospital, Heidelberg Victoria, Australia); James S. Olver (University of Melbourne. Deputy Director, General Hospital Psychiatry, Austin Health)

Series: Pharmacology – Research, Safety Testing and Regulation

Book Description: This volume brings together the clinical evidence for efficacy in these important conditions. Additionally, it explores in detail the pharmacokinetics, metabolism and mechanism of action of the drug. All medications have side effects associated with their use and duloxetine is no exception.

Hardcover ISBN: 978-1-53614-327-0
Retail Price: $160

Prescription Drugs: Global Perspectives, Long-Term Effects and Abuse Prevention

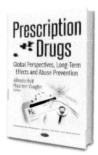

Editors: Alfredo Holt and Maureen Vaughn

Series: Pharmacology - Research, Safety Testing and Regulation

Book Description: In the first chapter, several different scenarios are described and surgical maneuvers for mitigating complications and improving outcomes in patient populations are examined.

Softcover ISBN: 978-1-53612-346-3
Retail Price: $82

Beta-Blockers: Physiological, Pharmacological and Therapeutic Implications

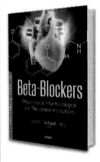

EDITOR: John R. Richards, M.D. (Department of Emergency Medicine, University of California, Davis School of Medicine, Sacramento, California, USA)

SERIES: Pharmacology - Research, Safety Testing and Regulation

BOOK DESCRIPTION: In the late 1950s, Sir James Black made a tremendous contribution to pharmacology and medicine with his discovery of â-blockers. After the first â-blockers became available in the 1960s, these drugs were noted to have beneficial effects in reducing morbidity and mortality from ischemic heart disease.

HARDCOVER ISBN: 978-1-53613-311-0
RETAIL PRICE: $230

Doxycycline: Medical Uses and Effects

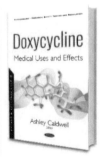

EDITOR: Ashley Caldwell

SERIES: Pharmacology – Research, Safety Testing and Regulation

BOOK DESCRIPTION: *Doxycycline: Medical Uses and Effects* opens with a personal account of experiments suggesting that doxycycline may play an important role in the fight against cancer and T-cell proliferation-related diseases.

SOFTCOVER ISBN: 978-1-53614-633-2
RETAIL PRICE: $82